PASSIONISTA

Ian Kerner, Ph.D.

PASSIONISTA

The Empowered Woman's Guide to Pleasuring a Man

(Previously published as
He Comes Next)

WILLIAM MORROW
An Imprint of HarperCollins*Publishers*

Hardcover edition published as HE COMES NEXT
FIRST PAPERBACK EDITION.

Designed by Kate Nichols
Illustrations by Naomi Pitcairn

Library of Congress Cataloging-in-Publication Data

Kerner, Ian.
Passionista: the empowered woman's guide to pleasuring a man /
Ian Kerner. —1st paperback ed.
p. cm.
Originally published: He comes next.
Includes bibliographical references.
ISBN 978-0-06-083439-5
1. Sex instruction for women.   2. Oral sex.   3. Male orgasm.   I. Title.

HQ46.K437 2008
613.9'6—dc22
2007038303

24 25 26 27 28 LBC 36 35 34 33 32

For Lisa,

my she in *She Comes First*

Contents

Part II: Techniques

Preface:
The Passionista on the Shaky Bridge

*Warning: This book is not recommended
for any woman with a fear of heights.*

ALLOW ME to explain.

If you ever happen to find yourself crossing the Capilano River in North Vancouver, Canada, you'll have two bridges to choose from. The first is definitely not for the faint of heart: A mere five feet wide and 450 feet long, the Capilano Canyon Suspension Bridge is constructed solely of plank and cable and sways perilously in the wind some 250 feet above the turbulent rocky tides—right out of a scene from Alfred Hitchcock's *Vertigo*. Your other choice? A solidly built anchored bridge that rests a mere ten feet above sea level.

In 1974, two well-known psychologists, Arthur Aron and Donald

Dutton, used these bridges as the focus of an ingenious experiment—one that sought to explore the mysterious nature of sexual attraction.

The two-part experiment went something like this: On day one, whenever an unaccompanied man ventured across the shaky bridge, he would find himself stopped midway by a beautiful young woman. She would introduce herself as a psychology researcher and then proceed to ask if he would mind participating in a brief survey.

On day two, the identical routine would be conducted by the same woman on the sturdy bridge.

Sounds pretty straightforward, right? But there was a little twist: When each of the men completed the survey, the young woman would hand him her phone number and tell him that he was free to call her later that evening for the results.

Unbeknownst to the subjects, the real study was not the answers the men gave to the survey, but what happened afterward. Aron and Dutton set out to examine which of the men gave the pretty psychologist a call and, more importantly, *why*. In other words, they were interested in studying not just what happened *on* the bridge, but how that affected what happened later. Would the excitement and exhilaration of being on the shaky bridge, versus the more mundane experience of being on the solid bridge, promote romantic attraction?

In technical terms, Aron and Dutton were testing a concept called "misattribution," also known as excitation transfer theory: Could lingering excitement from one situation—say, walking across a shaky bridge versus a stable one—intensify a subsequent emotional state? Or, to put it simply: Does adrenaline make the heart grow fonder?

The answer? Indeed, it does.

Not only did Aron and Dutton find that the men on the shaky bridge were more likely than their stable-bridge counterparts to call the woman later for results of the survey, but they were also *far more likely to ask her for a date!*

We'll come back to this experiment a little later when we talk about the roles that excitement and novelty play in stimulating our brain's natural "sex wiring," and I'll outline my "shaky bridge" approach to great sex. (Don't worry: It doesn't involve getting it on while bungee jumping—though that probably wouldn't hurt, accidents notwithstanding.)

Based on my experience working with couples, it's my wholehearted conviction that beneath the layers of linens that cover our conjugal beds, there lies a shaky bridge, ready and waiting for high-stakes action. Yet most of us spend our sex lives on the stable, sturdy one—often without realizing it. As your friendly neighborhood sex therapist, I'm here to help you take a monumental leap from one bridge to the other.

But before we shake things up, allow me to wax poetic for a moment on The Woman on the Shaky Bridge:

She is Dante's Beatrice and Gatsby's Daisy; she is Guinevere, Juliet, Helen, and Eurydice, to name a few.

You get the point. The woman on the shaky bridge is the stuff that dreams are made of, the gold from which love at first sight is wrought. She's sexy and exciting—the embodiment of desirability, the essence of allurement. She is a sexual muse: a passionista.

But believe it or not, the greatest asset of the Woman on the Shaky Bridge is not her beauty or her body; it's her brain. It's her knowledge of sexual psychology and her ability to apply it—*it's knowing which bridge to be on in the first place*, having the courage to cross it, and inspiring a guy to meet you in the middle.

My goal in these pages is far more ambitious than to provide you with a collection of hot sex tips and techniques. I want to give you more than just a way of a way of *doing*; I want to give you a vision: a way of *thinking* and *being*.

Regardless of your looks, body, or age; whether you're single or married; whether you're approaching date number three or 3,000, I want nothing less than to make *you* the passionista on the shaky bridge.

Let's start the journey.

Introduction:
The Best Sex He Never Had

GUYS LOVE TO TALK to me about sex. And I don't just mean in my office; I mean *everywhere*. I can't walk down the street without getting stopped: the UPS man, my super, my upstairs neighbor—hell, I know more about what turns on the guy behind the deli counter at my local grocery store than his own wife does.

One guy in particular, named Charlie, always makes me smile. He's a salesman for a pharmaceutical company, and we share an office suite, so I occasionally run into him at the coffee machine. With George Clooney looks, Charlie has a sex life that most men would envy. Every time I see him, he leans in close and whispers in hushed, enthusiastic tones: "Doc, last night I had the most *amazing* sex of my life. She was *incredible*. Can I just tell you—?"

That's when I have to cut him off and excuse myself. After all, I have a life to live. I have patients, deadlines, a wife, and two sons—if I indulged every guy who wanted to stop and talk to me about sex, I'd never get anything done.

But once I made the decision to write a book about male sexuality, that's exactly what I did: I stopped and listened to every guy who wanted to talk to me about sex. In fact, I sought them out. Traveling on my book tour, I met men of all stripes. And every time I sat down with a guy for the first time, I always began with the same lead-in: "Tell me about *the best sex* you ever had."

And boy did I get an earful. Not only did I hear about the best sex they ever had, but also, more importantly, I heard about the best sex they *never* had—experiences they always desired and fantasized about but were afraid to share with their partners for fear of offending or seeming weird. I heard the question "am I normal?" so many times that I'm now convinced that when it comes to sex, the *only* thing normal is that everyone's different.

To really get to know a guy, you practically have to wake up inside his skin, get inside his head, and know what it feels like to have a penis, with all the fantasies, desires, fears, and anxieties that go along with it. So think of Part I of *Passionista* as your own personal *Freaky Friday*—the closest you'll ever want to come to waking up in a guy's skin and knowing what truly makes him tick.

Great sex isn't about techniques or knowing what works; it's about knowing how and why it works. From the latest findings on the brain-chemistry of desire to the physiology of snuggling to a review of the three different types of erections all men experience, I'll take you on a guided tour of his body, brain, and mind that will leave no nook or cranny unexplored.

As for Part II, remember when I warned you that this book wasn't for women with a fear of heights? As I'm sure you know, I wasn't talking about literal heights. I'm talking about reaching new heights in pleasure, intimacy, and erotic creativity. So, get ready to take a walk out on that shaky bridge and stir things up because in Part II we'll talk about tactics, techniques, and tips.

But let me be clear: *Passionista* is not an encyclopedia of sexual positions or a catalog. I'm not out to give you an all-in-one, blow-by-blow (sorry, I couldn't resist) reference guide, but rather a clear, concise, *achievable* vision of sexual pleasure, one in which each part forwards the action, and where the whole is greater than the sum of its parts.

Sexual pleasure goes beyond techniques and tactics. Our sexual identities—and the expression, gratification, and growth of these identities—is fundamental to our overall health and the success of our intimate relationships. If most of us live in a world where the best sex we ever had is the best sex we *never* had, then it is of little wonder that sexual problems are among the leading causes of divorce and relationship dissatisfaction.

At heart, *Passionista* is a natural extension of the feminist philosophy of my first book, *She Comes First*, one in which I encouraged men to make love with more than just their penises, but with their entire selves.

While a man's genitals are clearly at the epicenter of his experience of sexual pleasure, they can also serve as an impediment to a more fully embodied sexual experience. The penis is often the focal point of a man's sexual anxiety, stemming from issues such as size, stamina, and performance: "Am I big enough, am I *too* big, will I be able to get it up, will I be able to keep it up, what if I get off too soon, what if it takes too long?" And so forth, and so on.

Sex therapists call this condition "spectatoring"—a process in which a person anxiously watches his or her own engagement in the sexual event, rather than being fully immersed in the moment itself. Those most afflicted with this tendency will judge and evaluate their performance, even while it's happening. Some therapists believe that spectatoring is the primary cause of most sexual issues in men. As anthropologist Lionel Tiger wrote in *The Decline of Males,* "Intimacy becomes a performance art."

Now, I'm not saying that your typical guy "spectates" to the point of sexual disorder, but it's been my observation that most men suffer from it to a varying extent. In the same way a woman may lose an orgasm by fretting over how she looks during sex—whether she's wet enough, thin enough, too slow to climax, too loud, not loud enough—men's ability to experience sexual pleasure is similarly impaired by a self-conscious feeling of being watched, especially when the spectator turns out to be their harshest critic: themselves.

Male sexual anxiety is on the rise. This has much to do with the proliferation of porn, especially given its easy access through the Internet and its emergence into mainstream pop culture. With sex books on the market, like the Vivid Girls' *How to Have a XXX Sex Life* and *Porn Star Secrets of Sex,* one of the greatest things you can do for a guy is reassure him that he *doesn't* have to make love like a porn star to satisfy you. Now, more than ever, women need to take an active role in this mission to liberate men from their own oppressively high, unrealistic standards. That's because, in addition to porn, the pharmaceutical industry is targeting younger and younger men with erectile stimulants, such as Viagra, Levitra, and Cialis, and bombarding them with marketing messages that reinforce a penis-focused, intercourse-based vision of sex that preys on performance anxieties and breeds spectatoring.

As an article in the *New York Times* noted, "Many men take Viagra to offset the pressure they feel to perform perfectly in a hyper-sexualized age." Soon it won't just be a condom in a hopeful teenager's wallet; it'll be a condom and little blue pill. (Whenever I lecture at a university, I'm always amazed and disheartened by the show of hands when I ask how many guys in the audience pop Viagra on a regular basis recreationally. It's not because they need it, they boast proudly, but because it gives them a better hard-on. And isn't that what women want?!)

But as any woman will attest, just because a guy has a hard-on doesn't mean he knows what to do with it. And with the "rise" of Viagra, it looks like "hard times" ahead for the female orgasm—unless you set him straight and show him how to put the focus on his erection to bed.

Even though this is a book about pleasuring men, your pleasure remains a fundamental right and an essential part of sex. That's one of the main tenets of being a passionista. As best-selling author and zoologist Desmond Morris has written in his homage to the female body, *The Naked Woman*, "Every woman has a beautiful body—beautiful because it is the brilliant end-point of millions of years of evolution. It is loaded with amazing adjustments and subtle refinements that make it the most remarkable organism on the planet." Your pleasure is vital to his pleasure. It's not about what you do *to* him; it's about what you do *with* him.

The sex you give is only as good as the sex you get. In that sense, *Passionista* is as much about your enjoyment of sex as it is about his.

Feminists of the 1960s and 1970s fought hard to reclaim a woman's right to sexual pleasure and make feminism synonymous with sexual freedom and equality. Many of today's women were born into the spirit of sexual entitlement and have never known it any other way. Their struggle is not for the right to be sexual, but rather how to use it. Today's woman has choices, but what she does with them is another matter.

Meanwhile, today's man is waiting for answers. Faced with independent, sexually liberated women, masculinity is in a state of flux and up for grabs, as it were, which is why the double-punch of porn and Viagra is so persuasive—and dangerous. Says Dr. Derek C. Polonsky, a clinical psychiatrist and sex therapist at Harvard Medical School, "The script that many men follow is one that is tailor-made for increasing anxiety and isolation. . . . it is often based on the unrealistic portrayal of sexuality in movies, where there is a seamless progression through intensifying states of sexual arousal and breathless nonverbal passion, usually with the male directing the pace and at all times knowing exactly what will please his partner." But the good news is that now, more than ever, sex-scripts (the ways in which we make love) are ripe for revision, and that's why women must seize the opportunity to turn attitude into action. It's your turn to lead.

In the very first episode of *Sex and the City*, Carrie ruminates on whether, in an age when women often enjoy the same income, power, and success as men, can they also enjoy having sex like men? While my knee-jerk response is yes, of course, on second thought, I believe that today's woman can do better. Rather than having sex like a man, she can teach her man how to have sex like a woman: how to make sex more sensual, more intimate, more open and connected, and, ultimately, more pleasure focused for both.

In the preface, I spoke of the Passionista on the Shaky Bridge as a poetic ideal. But in reality, our sex lives are often far from perfect; they're rife with subtext, miscommunication, and ambiguity, as well as unspoken wants and guilty desires. That's why I keep a framed photo of the Capilano Canyon Suspension Bridge on my desk—not only to show my patients, but also to remind myself, as a man and as a husband, that I have to be willing to venture across that bridge too if I want to find the exciting woman at its center. It's all about meeting each other halfway and taking the journey together, one in which we never stop growing.

Pop Quiz

Feel free to read *Passionista* in whatever manner you find comfortable. However, if you're inclined to skip Part I and go straight to the techniques in Part II, then I ask you first to consider a few simple questions.

- What's the best sex toy money *can't* buy?
- What are the three types of erections all men experience?
- Is your guy faking it? That's right—*faking it*. How do you know for sure?
- How can a properly administered pelvic massage actually help to lengthen your partner's penis?
- If, as the poet Ogden Nash wrote, "Candy is dandy, but liquor is quicker," what are the brain's natural sex-stimulants, and how do you get them flowing?
- What's the difference between orgasm and ejaculation, and are the two inextricably linked?
- Do you know the difference between a "local" orgasm and a "global" one and how to stimulate the latter?

If you're unsure about any of these important questions, then, in the spirit of *She Comes First*, think about postponing *your* immediate gratification and read *Passionista* from start to finish.

Postscript

When I got back to New York from my national tour, I had almost forgotten about Charlie (the George Clooney "womanizer"). So, when I ran into him at the coffee machine and, on cue, he said, "Doc, last night I had the most *amazing* sex. She was *incredible*. Can I just tell you . . . ," I said yes and dragged him into my office to get the 411.

The first thing I learned about Charlie's sex life was that all the various women he'd gone on and on about were, in fact, one woman: his wife of nine years and the mother of their two children, with a third on the way.

Charlie never stopped being in love with his wife, and the sex, to this day, remains fantastic.

Want to know his secret?

I'll tell you.

But first . . .

Dear Ian

●●●●●●●●●●

Dear Ian,

Doesn't being a sex therapist take some of the awe and joy out of sex for you? After all, sex is more than just mechanics and positions (Insert A into B and twist until secure)—it's an expression of love. And isn't love ultimately mysterious and unknowable?

—Latitia, twenty-eight, advertising production manager

WHAT A GREAT QUESTION to help me frame my preliminary thoughts on male sexuality. The more I learn about the nature of love and its expression through sexual intimacy, the more I *am* in awe of it. But sometimes I think we use the concept "love is a mystery" to avoid responsibility for the hard work true intimacy entails. We live in a culture in dire need of sexual education.

The number two reason for divorce in this country, after financial conflict, is sexual dissatisfaction, and a crucial part of the problem is lack of communication and poor information. When it comes to talking about sex with a partner, breaking the ice is like breaking an iceberg, and all of us know what happened to the *Titanic*.

To give you a sense of my clinical philosophy, let me briefly explain how I approach a new patient or couple. Sex therapy generally follows a model called P-LI-SS-IT, which stands for permission, limited information, specific suggestions, and intensive therapy. First, a patient needs *permission* to confront an issue openly and safely with a therapist or counselor. Second, they need accurate *information*—ranging from physiological facts to psychological reactions—to tackle their problems. Next, they need *specific suggestions* to get them back on the road to sexual health. In some circumstances, they may also need *intensive therapy*, though most of the time the first three steps will do the trick.

I've adapted the P-LI-SS-IT model to accommodate my own working version, which I call the "See Me, Feel Me, Touch Me, Heal Me" approach to counseling. (Yes, I listened to The Who a lot growing up.) For counseling to succeed, a patient must, first and foremost, be seen. This is important when you consider how many people are leading lives of quiet desperation when it comes to personal relationships. Next, that individual must be felt. Their emotional turmoil must be communicated effectively and experienced by their partner. The third, and touchy, part takes the form of sex and intimacy assignments that are done at home and then discussed in subsequent sessions. All of this must occur before a person can *even begin* the process of healing. So, to answer my reader's question, love *is* indeed mysterious. Sexual ignorance, however, is not. It's a function of laziness, prejudice, and fear. The more we learn about sex, the more there is to appreciate, understand, and savor.

Hey, just because we hit an iceberg doesn't mean we have to go down with the ship!

PASSIONISTA

PART

The Male Body

ONE

Beneath His Armor:
Inside the Male Body

O KAY, PASSIONISTAS, picture this: A guy gets up in the middle of the night to go to the bathroom and slowly winds his way through a dark room cluttered with furniture. One hand is out in front of him as he gropes for the bathroom door and light switch, but what do you think the other hand is doing?

Protecting his genitals.

Sounds obvious, right? Men protect their privates. And why shouldn't we? After all, nobody wants the family jewels getting chipped.

But what if I told you that this idea of self-protection goes far beyond a simple reflex and is, rather, the key to fathoming the inner recesses and dark corners of male sexuality?

Allow me to elaborate. Men's genitals grow outward. From an early age on, boys intuitively protect them. But over time, this instinctive desire to protect manifests itself as a permanent sense of inwardness, a physical "pulling in" that ultimately extends to the entire pelvic area. (If you don't believe me, the next time you're on a dance floor, take a look at the guys around you. They're all arms and legs, as if they're doing the "Dance of the Missing Middle.")

Over the years, I've talked to countless physical therapists, chiropractors, as well as dance and yoga instructors, all of whom concur that the adult male pelvis is frequently in a state of tension. All of these professionals, in one way or another, work with guys to help them "open up"—sometimes to help manage back pain, sometimes in the course of facilitating recovery from an injury, and other times just to get them through that first dance at their wedding reception without looking like Frankenstein.

One of my goals in this book is to help you open up your guy's pelvis, so he can experience sex in a way that's less inhibited and more sensual and exciting.

But this sense of pulling in is more than just physical. Men are shrouded in layers of "protection"—physical, emotional, psychological—that find a nexus in the pelvis, but permeate throughout the body and mind. In this sense, every man is a knight in shining—or not-so-shining—armor.

Now I know what you're thinking: *Hold on a minute. Protection? Please! I'm the one that could use some protecting—every time he pushes my head down and expects me to open wide and say, "Ahhhh."*

But that's *exactly* what I'm talking about. For most men, sex begins and ends with the penis and rarely extends beyond it. From a fear of having his testicles rough-housed to sensitivity around the perineum (the area between the testicles and anus that is rife with nerve endings and shields the male G-spot) to a nobody-touches-me-down-there attitude about his butt, the male experience of sex is one that's controlled, circumscribed, and the living embodiment of uptight.

Some of these protections are physiological and involuntary—like the "cremaster reflex," which is triggered when you touch his inner thigh. The testicles literally pull up and in. But many are largely psychological in nature.

The journey to, and through, manhood is very much a journey of learning to stay in control. As R. Louis Schultz, M.D., wrote in his seminal book, forgive the pun, *Out in the Open: The Complete Male Pelvis*:

> To live in society, we all require a degree of control. Too much control, however, and we can become automatons. Control is always being right. Control is not letting your feelings influence your life. Control is not letting the joy of life be a goal. Control is not expressing your feelings. Control is being neutral or neuter. Control is not being sensual. Control is lessening the enjoyment of sex. Control is not being aware or responsive to the feelings of others, since you are not aware of your own feelings. Control is always being on an even emotional plane.

I quoted this passage at length because, even though Dr. Schultz's astute observations are based on his experiences as a physician and deep tissue massage expert, I've too often heard in counseling these exact complaints from women about men: "He's disconnected from his feelings;" "He won't let go; he keeps everything inside;" "We have sex, but we don't make love;" "He won't talk about sex; he walks away the minute I bring up the conversation;" and so on and so on.

Dr. Schultz continues on the subject of control and its physical manifestations: "To achieve such control is not to feel, to become numb. This can apply to the entire body and is especially true in the anogenital region. Protection begins by pulling in the offending penis and anus."

Later in our discussion, when we talk about the male mind, this area—the anogenital region, or complete pelvis as Dr. Schultz has dubbed it—often figures heavily in sexual desires and fantasies. Although it's heavily guarded and sometimes taboo, the pelvis is ultimately a region that signals abandon and capitulation, an area of letting go and surrender to which men want to succumb, but are timorous. Beyond the penis is a whole new world of erotic pleasure to discover and explore. But, unless he's a Chinese contortionist, it's completely virgin territory, the physical equivalent of the Forbidden City.

So let's take a look at the complete pelvis, and why—for both

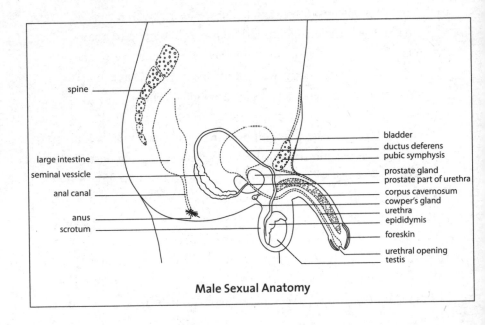

Male Sexual Anatomy

physical and psychological reasons—its various parts are subject to layers of protection, and how you, as a passionista, can start to unlock those areas.

Head Case

Commencing our journey at the penis, the part that gets the most attention is the glans, or head. This soft, fleshy area swells during arousal and is replete with sensitive nerve endings. From the ridge of the corona to the underside of the frenulum (which many men consider their "sexual sweet spot"), the glans is indubitably the most physically sensitive part of a man's body.

Like a woman's clitoris, the glans is incredibly sensitive to touch, especially after orgasm or in the early stages of arousal. The glans is the area that most men stimulate heavily, even exclusively, during masturbation. For some men, their pursuit of pleasure never extends

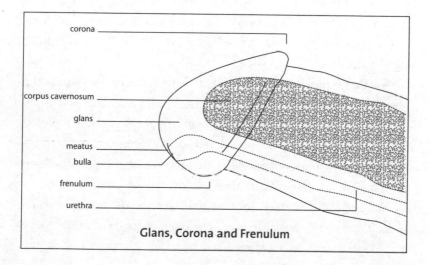

corona

corpus cavernosum

glans

meatus

bulla

frenulum

urethra

Glans, Corona and Frenulum

beyond the head of their penis. As author Sally Tisdale wrote in her book, *Talk Dirty to Me: An Intimate Philosophy of Sex*, "Male sexuality seems different from mine fundamentally because nothing need be involved but the head and shaft of the penis, no other part of the body need be troubled, touched, undressed, or soiled. . . ."

But the glans, by dint of its very sensitivity, is also a protected area, both physically and psychologically. And when it comes to physical stimulation of the glans, the complaints of men are not dissimilar to those of women, who often protest about guys who make a mad rush for the clitoral head. As one woman told me, "Every time he goes down on me, it's like the running of the bulls at Pamplona— I just want to get the hell out of his way!" But women aren't the only ones who get rushed. Here, from the annals of persecuted penises:

"She milked me like I was a cow!"

"She bit into my cock like it was a stick of pepperoni!"

"Watch the teeth; *watch the teeth!*"

One guy, a police officer who's seen more than his fair share of mayhem, said of his wife's oral abilities, "I'm telling you, I'm more scared of her blow jobs than I am of rushing a crack house. At least in the crack house, I can suit up. What I really need is a bulletproof vest for my dick!"

Another type of protection that finds its focus in the glans is the fear of premature ejaculation (PE), also known as rapid ejaculation. Almost every guy struggles to some degree with PE. It's been reported that PE is *three times* more prevalent in the United States than erectile disorder. Countless reports cite that the anxiety of ejaculating too quickly significantly decreases men's enjoyment of sex.

Sex and the City star Kim Cattrall wrote in her book, *Satisfaction*, "Premature ejaculators were the bane of my existence." And I can assure you from a guy's perspective that it's no fun being the

Q UESTION TO MEN: *"Have you ever named your penis, and/or what did/would you name it?*
ANSWER: Spike, Godzilla, King Kong, Pee-Wee, Sea Monkey, Nervous Nelly, Iron John, the Little Engine That Could (n't).

QUESTION TO WOMEN: *If you could, what would you name your guy's penis?*
ANSWER: Speedy, Zippy, Weary, Wrinkly, Lazy, Woody (as in Allen—neurotic and hesitant), the little Engine That "Shoulda, Coulda, Woulda."

bane of any woman's existence, especially when it comes to sexual performance or Kim Cattrall. While we're inundated with commercials for Viagra and its competitors, and impotence seems to have gone mainstream (with its media-friendly metamorphosis into erectile disorder), rapid ejaculators still suffer in silence.

What it all comes down to is that the sensitive glans is an area of conflict. There's nothing more enjoyable than having it stimulated, but all too often, the pleasures prove nerve wracking and overwhelming. As Dr. Alex Comfort wrote of fellatio in *The New Joy of Sex,* "A few men can't take even the shortest genital kiss before ejaculating."

Bad masturbation habits don't help matters. By focusing on the head during self-pleasuring, men have hard-wired themselves for rapid ejaculation, which can lead to a lifetime of sexual failures. I've counseled guys who have been so distraught over PE that they'd rather not date at all or they've ended meaningful relationships with women—often without even telling them why.

Chronic sufferers of PE have been known to wear double condoms, imbibe alcohol, apply numbing agents, run baseball

Dear Ian
  How do I deal with a guy who suffers from premature ejaculation without bruising his ego?

  —Maisy, thirty-one

Follow this three-step process—Please, Squeeze, At Ease—to help him step on the brakes and savor the trip:

STEP 1: PLEASE

If your guy suffers from PE, you don't have to get into a whole angst-ridden conversation about it; in fact, you can work on his problem without him ever knowing you know it's a problem. And you can make it a whole lot of fun.

Tell your guy you want him to experience the ecstatic pleasures of male multiple orgasms: You're going to bring him as close to the edge as possible, but he needs to help you by letting you know when he's about to go over. By using manual and oral stimulation to bring him close to the point of ejaculatory inevitability, but not past it, he will experience one or two pleasurable orgasmic contractions, which will expel some of the sexual tension that has built up in his pelvic region, release some blood from his penis, and slow him down.

STEP 2: SQUEEZE

Once you've done some pleasing, it's time for some squeezing. Apply firm pressure with your thumb and forefinger, and focus the pressure on the urethra, the tube running along the underside of the penis. Squeeze right below the head of his penis. This technique, developed by Masters and Johnson, pushes blood out of the penis and suppresses the ejaculatory response.

STEP 3: AT EASE

After you've given him a good squeeze, back off of his penis and go back to hugging and kissing, and focus on stimulating other body parts. Give it a good thirty to sixty seconds before you return to any form of direct genital stimulation. Not only does the "at ease" period let him relax and cool down, it's also a chance for him to practice some pleasing on you.

Rapid ejaculators are typically very anxious about wanting their partners to experience orgasms and are generally all too happy to give you manual and oral stimulation or introduce a sex toy into the action. It's all part of the sexual courtesy that was at the heart of my book *She Comes First* and part of a philosophy that allows a rapid ejaculator to develop confidence and control while simultaneously pleasuring you. Take the emphasis off of simultaneous orgasms and focus on serial orgasms: one after the other, yours first.

statistics, even think about dead people—anything to reduce the pleasure. But, in truth, their efforts are misguided. Rather than reduce pleasure, men should be encouraged to increase and distribute pleasure—to extend the sexual experience to areas beyond the glans.

The First Cut Is the Deepest

In uncircumcised men, the glans is covered with a prepuce, or foreskin, from which it emerges during arousal. Circumcision, a common practice in the United States, but not elsewhere in the world, is increasingly becoming a matter of debate, with many likening it to genital mutilation.

There are those traditionalists—often members of the medical establishment—who maintain that the foreskin is an unimportant, functionless flap of skin that inhibits hygiene and can potentially cause infection in both men and women, as well as increase vulnerability to sexually transmitted infections (STIs).

But another school of thought holds that the foreskin plays a significant role in both sexual pleasure and hygiene. The foreskin is filled with nerve endings, and any uncircumcised male will tell you that stimulating it is a source of tremendous pleasure.

But for most uncircumcised men in the United States, the foreskin often creates an extra layer of protection that is entirely unwanted. Uncircumcised males are sensitive to their foreskin's strangeness and often encounter confusion, or even disgust, from both men and women. As an example, one woman told me that when she first encountered a former boyfriend's foreskin, she joked, "Now what the hell am I supposed to do with *that*?" From that time onward, the poor guy experienced erectile disorder and was unable to get an erection in her presence.

* * * * * * * * * *

Dear Ian,

So, I was about to go down on my new boyfriend for the first time when I was stopped in my tracks by a foreskin. Hel-lo! I've only been with normal guys before, and it kind of freaks me out. What should I do?

—Jenny, twenty-six, legal secretary

First of all, please be advised that while circumcision is prevalent in North America, it's much less common in Europe and other culturcs. So taking a global perspective, it's really far more "normal" for a guy *not* to be circumcised.

Also know that the foreskin can play a pivotal role in both his pleasure and *yours*. The foreskin is filled with sensitive receptors that turn him on. And when it retracts behind the glans, it creates a wider ridge that many women find especially stimulating during sex. Some women refer to the bundled-up foreskin as a built-in "G-spot stimulator."

Also, uncircumcised men are usually hypersensitive about hygiene, so know that he's probably cleaner than most guys. (I once did a survey of women, "Which matters more, a big penis or a clean penis?" Clean won hands [*and* mouth] down.)

But it's all right to tell him that you've never been with a guy with a foreskin before. You probably won't be the first. As a passionista, just remember to express yourself in a positive, constructive manner and know that not only will his foreskin not hinder great sex, but also it will probably enhance it. As one woman told me, "A foreskin is the best sex toy money *can't* buy."

* * * * * * * * * *

Shafted

Continuing our journey of the penis, the shaft is the middle section and consists of three cylindrical spheres of soft tissue. In his clever book, *Talking Cock*, author Richard Herring dubs the corpus cavernosum, the two larger cylinders, "'the lung of desire' because it almost seems to 'breathe in' blood during arousal. And it holds that breath until its work is done. It's not a 'hollow chamber' as the translated

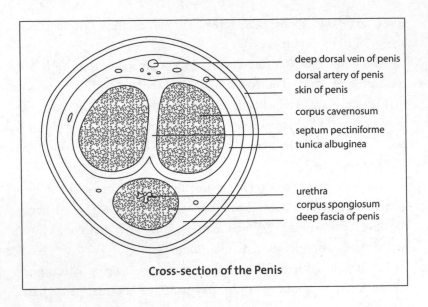

deep dorsal vein of penis
dorsal artery of penis
skin of penis

corpus cavernosum

septum pectiniforme
tunica albuginea

urethra
corpus spongiosum
deep fascia of penis

Cross-section of the Penis

Latin would have us believe. It is full of sound and fury. It's a sensational, expanding hive of blood."

Think of it as the hydraulics of desire. A system of "valves" enables blood to be retained in the penis and then allows blood to be expelled post-ejaculation, which returns it to a flaccid state.

. . . .

Does Size Matter?

In many men, the penile shaft is the focal point of anxieties around size. We already know that many guys worry that they're too small, but there are also some guys who worry about being too large. Penis size plays a significant role in performance anxiety in men of all shapes and sizes.

So, does size really matter? It's a subjective question. It matters if it matters to you. The clitoris, located at the surface of the vulva, is the powerhouse of the female orgasm, so technically deep penetration is not necessary for a woman to experience orgasm. However, the G-spot is reached inside the vagina, and a clitoral orgasm enhanced by G-spot stimulation would require penetration either with a penis, hand, or sex toy. But as the G-spot is only one to three inches inside the vaginal entrance, nearly any penis will do, unless the guy has a micro-penis—a truly "teenie-weenie"—a condition which, according to BBC News, afflicts one in 200 men, with a penis less than two and a half inches in length, erect. In fact, when you consider that virtually all of the sensitive nerve endings that contribute to the female orgasm are located within the first inch or so of the vaginal entrance, girth (thickness) matters more than length. Later, we'll talk about techniques to naturally lengthen his penis via pelvic massage.

Looks are often deceiving. A small, nonerect penis will often double in size when erect. And while most heterosexual women enjoy the physical sensation and/or emotional closeness of penile penetration, because the vagina is actually a compressed tube that "tents" during arousal and wraps itself around the penis, size matters less than is generally assumed. But sex goes beyond the mechanics of orgasm production. It's a physical, psychological, and emotional experience, all of which affects how a particular woman will ultimately feel about penis size.

Many guys seem to assume that having a big penis is tantamount to being a good lover or, conversely, that having a small penis dooms you to the sexual sidelines. When push ultimately comes to shove, the majority of women feel that bigger does not *automatically* equal better. Much the way men may regard a woman's breasts as more or less erotic depending on size and shape, penis size, like breast size,

WHAT OTHER WOMEN SAY ABOUT SIZE

These days, what matters most is that it works. More and more, a good man is hard to find, or should I say a *hard* man is GOOD to find!"

"I don't mind if it's short, but hopefully it's also thick."

"It's all about a good fit. But that depends on the person more than the size of his dick. The fit has to be emotional and physical."

"If you love the man, then you love his penis."

"Size is irrelevant. Because most men don't know what to do with it, anyway."

"I like guys with small dicks because they work harder. Guys with big dicks are lazy."

"The great thing about the vagina is it's flexible—one size fits all!"

"Most guys don't last enough for me to really notice one way or the other."

has nothing to do with the actual physiology of orgasm or the propensity for sexual and sensual pleasure.

For many guys, penis size is really more a matter of vanity than a genuine concern for female pleasure. Like a fancy sports car or a nifty Rolex, it reinforces a sense of masculinity. And unlike women, who are likely to have honest conversations with other women about breast size and insecurities therein, men rarely, if ever, have a heart-to-heart about their penises. All a woman needs to do is look around to know that she lives in a world populated by breasts of all shapes and sizes. But when it comes to a guy worrying how he measures up, he doesn't have much to go on, unless he sneaks a peak in the locker room or at the urinal, at the risk of getting caught (and potentially beaten up). This means that guys tend to get much of their feedback about penis size from porn and the awfully "tall tales" of other men.

Also consider the fact that when a guy looks down at his own penis, the angle is likely to make him look smaller than he actually is, and it's easy to understand why, from pumps to pills, there's a massive market for all sorts of phony penis-enlargement products.

While I have yet to meet a woman who has suffered from penis envy, there seem to be plenty of *guys* who fall prey to this tendency. So perhaps Freud was onto something after all, given that he was just a man who, like most men, walked through life primarily flaccid. From surreptitiously checking out one another's members to envying the long-johns depicted in porn to ancient erotic renderings of exaggerated phalluses, men have long measured and compared their alleged virility based on penis size and turgidity.

And for those women who have chanced to ponder what it would be like to have "one of those things," here are a few "Member Musings" from other passionistas:

"If I had a penis, I'd pee standing up and wouldn't worry about whipping it out in a dark alley or behind a tree."

"I'd donate sperm."

"I'd make my boyfriend go down and swallow!"

"It would be interesting to penetrate, rather than be penetrated."

"I'd rule the world!"

"I'd make Dick Cheney squeal like a pig!"

In many cases, the issue of size comes up when a man is too big. Many women panic at the sight of a big penis and worry about

Dear Ian,

My boyfriend keeps saying he knows he has a small cock and apologizing for it, or he makes little self-deprecating remarks, and the truth is he does have a small penis. Whenever he makes a comment, I just act like I didn't hear him, but it only makes matters worse. Next time he goes on and on about his small penis, what should I do?

—Liz, twenty-eight, retail clothing buyer

Ask most women, and they will tell you in no uncertain terms that, when it comes to their beloved joysticks, men make far too much of far too little. In short, perhaps I should rephrase, men place way too much stock in penis size. In a recent survey I did of college guys, I asked, "If you could ask your girlfriend anything about your sex life, what would it be?" I was sure they'd want to know if she'd ever faked it, but do you know what the number one response was? "How does my dick measure up to other guys she's been with?"

As a woman, you can't underestimate just how much of a guy's sexual identity is wrapped around his penis. So, let me turn the question around: Does it bother *you* that he has a small penis? The truth is that whenever I talk to women who complain about their guy's lowly lower measurement, once we get around to discussing the real issues, the problem is rarely about *his* size, but rather *her* lack of orgasmic fulfillment. Whether you're satisfied or dissatisfied with your guy's size, you need to reframe the conversation to focus on quality, not quantity.

I've certainly met plenty of women who have broken up with a guy because of sexual dissatisfaction, but I've never met a woman who left a guy solely because of inadequate penis size. You know there's an old joke that goes, "A bastard is a guy who makes love to you with a three-inch penis and then kisses you good-bye with a six-inch tongue." This is just one more way of saying that there's more to sex than penis size. My advice is that the next time he makes a joke about his size, use it as a launching-point for some genuine communication. Ask him why he cares so much about his size. If he says it's because he wants to pleasure you or that he believes size is related to pleasure, take the opportunity to set him straight. As one woman I know told her husband, who was insecure about his size, "Look, yours isn't the only penis I've known, but it's the only one that's been worth knowing."

If that's still not enough, for those on the small side, it's been estimated that one to three inches of the penis is typically pulled into the perineum: The tighter the pelvic area, the more likely that the muscles in his perineum are pulling on his penis and drawing it into the body. When a man's pelvis is opened up through relaxation, breathing, and massage, all of which we will discuss later, it may actually lengthen his penis!

getting hurt. In some cases, it actually *can* lead to injury. Rarely does this mean you can't have sex with him, but it does mean taking it more slowly, making sure you're amply aroused, keeping plenty of lubrication on hand(s), and using a position like side-by-side, where you can easily hold and guide his penis. One female patient of mine was so afraid of the size of her fiancé's penis that she thought she might call off the wedding. What made the situation worse was that her girlfriends teased her about it and told her they'd kill to be in her shoes. But it's a genuine anxiety and one that's likely to be more damning to sexual relations than concerns over small penis size.

Dear Ian,

My boyfriend won't let me get on top during sex because he's afraid I'm going to "break" his penis? Is that even possible?

—Tania, thirty-six, attorney

Yes, believe it or not, it *is* possible to break one's penis, though highly unlikely. (Interestingly, male anxiety over breaking one's penis is far more prevalent than actual occurrences.)

Broken penises usually happen when an erect penis is thrust against a harder object, like a pelvic bone, for example. You'll know if he's broken his penis because you'll hear a "cracking" sound; he'll lose his erection, and his penis will bend to one side or the other. If it were to happen, he would need immediate medical attention and possibly even surgery—all in all, not a fun visit to the emergency room.

I have yet to meet any man who has ever actually broken his penis, though I have consulted with men who were born with Peyronie's disease, a congenital condition that causes a curvature of the penis due to fibrosis (hardened tissue). I have heard of only one case of a broken penis, where the woman, far larger and heavier than her sexual partner, pounced on her boyfriend with reckless abandon in a female-superior position and succeeded in fracturing his member. Needless to say, after an embarrassing trip to the ER and proper healing, the couple was less energetic in their romps.

As far as sex positions and broken penises go, the female-superior position is one of the least likely to land him in a penis splint (yes, they often need to "set" a broken penis) because most of the pressure (and pleasure) is a function of rubbing the clitoris against his pelvic bone. But if he's nervous about the position, start in the standard missionary or side-to-side position and let him penetrate you fully and then *gently* roll on top.

. . . .

Going South: The Road Less Traveled

Continuing our journey down the shaft of the penis toward the abdomen, we now reach the scrotum, which contains the testicles, or testes.

Typically, the left testicle hangs lower than the right because the left side descends first during birth. Approximately 75 percent of men hang to the left (although clearly this lefty disposition doesn't translate at the polls).

And talk about central air-conditioning: When exposed to heat, the scrotum loosens and pushes away from the body; but when exposed to cold, the scrotum pulls into the body and tightens.

Sexual arousal also causes the testicles to be pulled up into the body to protect them during sex. As mentioned earlier, if you want

From the Annals of Terrorized Testes:

"She gobbled up my balls like she was sucking dumplings!"

"Don't squeeze; caress!"

"Focus on the scrotum—the skin—not the testicles. Tickle, graze, nibble, pinch lightly."

"Every time my girlfriend touches my balls, I start to have a panic attack. It feels great, but it's also torture."

to test the cremasteric muscles, touch his inner thigh and just watch his testicles run for the scrotal hills.

From the scrotum, we continue our journey deeper into protected areas—hot-zones that abut (no pun intended) the taboo. The perineum contains the root of the penis.

Positioned between the scrotum and the anus, this area is sometimes called the "t'aint" because "it t'aint one or the other." But regardless of what it t'aint, it is most definitely an area rife with nerve endings and erectile tissue that swells during arousal with the infusion of blood to the pelvic area. It's also possible to stimulate the prostate—known as the male G-spot—through a perineal massage (that is, if he'll let you). With the scrotum to the north and the anus to the south, this area is typically more heavily guarded than Guantanamo Bay.

He Has Kegels Too

Both men and women have a PC (pubococcygeus) muscle, which is responsible for the health of the pelvis.

Exercising this muscle regularly will *naturally* help to prolong sex and allow him to distinguish better between orgasm and ejaculation and lead to a potentially more intense climax. As men age, they sometimes complain of orgasms that are less intense and pleasurable. One reason for this loss is the steady weakening of the PC muscle. That should be motivation enough. So the next time he heads off for the gym, tell him that weight lifting isn't the only exercise he should be doing.

If he wants some guidance on how to do them, tell him to practice by first stopping the flow of urine midstream—that will help him locate the muscle.

From there, he should do reps of kegels, gradually increasing the overall amount, as well as the length of time he holds the contraction. He can do them anywhere, but sometimes it's fun to practice them together.

When you're having intercourse, you'll both benefit from stronger kegels: He'll be able to last longer, and you'll feel it against your G-spot when he does them inside you. And remember that your kegels will feel great on him, particularly if you squeeze them while he's pulling out of you or, even better, having sex that involves mutual squeezing, rather than thrusting.

Butt Why?

Like the perineum, the anal entrance is rich with nerve endings and is a source of tremendous pleasure, but it's also protected (to say the least). Think of it as the *Heart of Darkness* of male sexuality. Mess around with him back there, and he's likely to get as loopy as Marlon Brando in *Apocalypse Now*.

The prostate gland is a walnut-size gland that lies below the urinary bladder and produces prostatic fluid. The white, sticky fluid forms most of the volume of semen and serves as its delivery mechanism.

The prostate is also a source of pleasure, one that can be stimulated through anal touch. Often called the male G-spot, I prefer to call it the *P-spot*, as in protected rather than prostate. If you and your partner want to enjoy this intense nugget of pleasure, you will

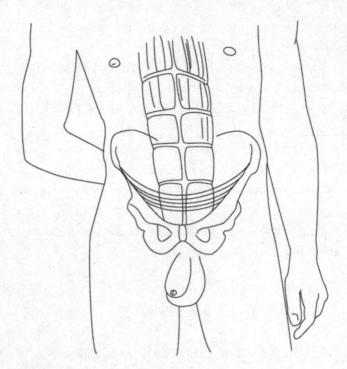

Rectus Abdominus, aka "the Six-Pack"

have to travel about one to three inches inside his rectum toward the front of his body (his stomach). For less intrusive pleasures, you can also stimulate the prostate externally through perineal massage.

Beyond the anus, there's the entire buttocks and the gluteus maximus muscles that run through them, which are often tight with tension. Additionally, there are bands of fibrous tissue (rectus ambdominus), aka the *"six-pack,"* situated beneath the abdomen in the groin area. As Dr. Louis Schultz observed in *Out in the Open: The Complete Male Pelvis*, these bands form a sort of interior jock strap, which, when overly tight, can restrict oxygen from reaching the area and contribute to a numbed sensation, inhibited arousal, erectile disorder, and less intense orgasms.

When exploring the male body, it's important to look beyond his penis and consider the entire pelvic region. In most sex, the penis drives, if not drags, the other parts along for the ride, which are left overly tense, or flaccid, and somewhat desensitized. Through a combination of factors, both physiological and psychological, the male compulsion to protect or guard this area can hobble sexual experience. By opening up the pelvis and engaging his entire pleasure platform, you can help him enjoy a heightened "out-of-body" sexual and sensual experience very much rooted *in his body.*

Male Sexual Response:
A Protected Process

WHENEVER I talk to men about their adult anxieties and sexual issues, invariably the subject shifts back to memories from their teenage years: embarrassing erections, troublesome wet dreams, and masturbation traumas. Many of the men grew up with brothers and sisters stealing precious moments of privacy, or with intrusive mothers banging at the bathroom door, demanding to be let in or berating them for stained sheets or underwear. No matter what your partner's personal experiences, his discovery of arousal's fierce hold and irrepressible timing no doubt caused him some trauma, embarrassment, and hardship during critical points in his psychosexual development. Hormonally driven cravings are often experienced as uncontrollable urges, from boyhood through early manhood, an unwieldly force to be managed stealthfully and quickly, rather than a source of joyous self-exploration.

Although the process of arousal, also known as sexual response, is a nuanced one, it's typically experienced as a mad rush to orgasm. The focus is on destination, rather than journey, and what should be appreciated and savored is often consumed ravenously like a condemned man's last meal.

As reinforced by masturbation, the male process of sexual response is often incompatible with a woman's. The differences manifest in the relationships we form. Some guys embrace the challenge and recalibrate their sexual behavior to mesh with their partners' needs. Others wallow in happy ignorance, owing to a partner's fear of rejection and consequent willingness to fake it. Then there are those who can't disabuse themselves of their adolescent fantasies, who retreat into porn-centric safety, denouncing any woman who cannot achieve orgasm through intercourse as frigid, unsexy, or aberrant.

Many men end up developing a sexual shorthand with their partners, a sex script that offers the path of least resistance to consistent gratification, one that reduces them to sexual automatons in which sex is familiar and routine. The orgasms may even be simultaneous, but they are emotionally and creatively hollow, no better in qualitative terms than the sexual release each partner could have had on their own. This is the world of the lonely orgasm.

But it doesn't have to be this way. By understanding the process of male sexual response, you can imbue it with spontaneity and unpredictability.

Desire

Sexuality researchers Masters and Johnson determined that the human sexual response cycle consists of four distinct stages: excitement, plateau, orgasm, and resolution.

But experts concur that there's another stage as well, one that overpowers the others: desire.

Desire is the most mercurial and mysterious of all the phases. In fact, when Masters and Johnson first defined the sexual response cycle, they didn't even include desire. One of the reasons for this is that desire and excitement (often used interchangeably with the term "arousal") are closely interlinked, especially in men. Give a guy an erection, and he wants to use it; hence the success of Viagra and other erectile stimulants, such as Cialis and Levitra. Stimulating arousal or excitement often stimulates desire itself.

So though there may be some truth to the statement that men are more easily aroused than women, don't fall prey to the assumption that guys are walking hard-ons, always ready for action. In fact, contrary to clichés, it's been my experience in working with couples with mismatched libidos that the partner with the lower sex drive is often the guy, so much so that I would say that low male desire is a silent epidemic, with sex-starved women often suffering in confusion and silent desperation.

In the next chapter, I'll specifically discuss the brain chemistry of the mating process, and why a loss of desire (relative to the infatuation phase) is a perfectly natural and ultimately manageable part of a healthy and fulfilling love life. But in a world wrought with clichés about male sexuality—"men are dogs; they'll screw anything"—the worst thing a woman can do is take desire for granted and assume he *should* want you just because, well, *he has a penis!*

A Bird in the Hand . . .

I often deal with women who are frustrated by the fact that their husband or boyfriend claims to have no interest in sex, but then they catch him masturbating. They feel betrayed and lied to: "How could he say he has no desire when he masturbates? Clearly he has an interest in sex, just not with me, *right?*"

Wrong. The fact that he's masturbating is a really positive sign: It means he still has a libido. He hasn't lost interest in sex; it just means your relationship needs some sexual maintenance, a tune-up, perhaps a fuel injection. With a little creativity and a lot of communication, you can breathe new life into your tired old sex routines by learning how to explore what turns him and you on together (more of this to come in Part II).

The truth is that when you fell in love, there were some very potent chemicals fueling the process and making desire a no-brainer. Now you have to work at it. But with that work (which is actually a whole lot of fun) comes a deepening of your relationship as well as a potentially more exciting, dynamic, and varied experience of sex. It may not be the euphoric, chemical-addled sex of infatuation, but that doesn't mean it won't be better or at least different.

For instance, I meet so many couples in their fifties and sixties who insist that the sex they're having now is better than ever before. Sure, they're the first to admit that sex has changed. But they also say that sex has become more creative and tender, less orgasm driven, more sensual, and ultimately intimate. (Some of this has to do with the fact that as men age, their testosterone levels decrease, while estrogen levels increase. So he's naturally discovering a softer side of sex.) The men who are the happiest are the ones who ultimately accept and embrace these natural changes and discover new paths in their sexual journeys.

Regardless of age, people change. Relationships change. Why should sex stay the same?

Desire is the launch-pad for the process of sexual response. But desire is more than just a starting point. It's the beginning, middle, and end of sex (and all the little steps in between), as well as the erotic glue between sexual encounters. Desire doesn't just give rise to sex; desire is borne of sex as well.

Excitement

Now that we're beyond the murky depths of desire, the road ahead becomes a bit more straightforward (albeit "wobbly" at times). In men, genital stimulation often causes an erection within a few seconds.

Did you know that all men experience three different types of erections? Count 'em: three.

The first type, produced by erotic stimuli, is considered a psychogenic erection, or what I like to think of as a "brain erection." Men also experience reflex erections as a result of direct genital stimulation, what I like to think of as a "body erection." And finally, they experience spontaneous nocturnal erections during REM cycles, explaining why guys are often into morning sex—they wake up in the midst of a nocturnal erection.

It's worth understanding each of these different erections

because all three play a role in arousal. As an example, when men become bored with sex, it's often due to a lack of fresh psychogenic stimuli within the relationship—in other words, a loss of erotic creativity.

Reflex erections are caused by physical stimulation of nerves in the genital area, initiating the first part of a reflex circuit and continuing to the lower spine. Once received and sent back to the erectile tissue in the penis, the circuit is completed and voilà! Enter the hard-on. Sometimes a man can be so depressed or stressed out that he's closed off to both psychogenic and reflex stimuli. That said, he will often still wake up in the morning with a nocturnal erection, and I advise women to use this as a starting point. Hey, if he's got it, use it. As we discussed a little earlier, sex can be a springboard for increasing desire. An exciting sexual encounter today is what tomorrow's desire-based fantasies are made of.

For this reason, I sometimes counsel patients to take advantage of the reflex erection and to focus simply on physical stimulation, as there's truth in the idea that sex begets more sex. Some men just need to be physically jumpstarted, so, as per the slogan for Nike, just do it.

As simple as it sounds, one of the best ways to break out of a sex rut is to have sex. This is especially true of men, where studies of the brain during sexual stimulation, using a technique called positron emission tomography (PET), reveal that men appear to focus significantly more on the sensations transmitted from the genitals to the brain than do women. As Gert Holstege of the University of Groningen told the European Society of Human Reproduction and Embryology conference in Copenhagen, "This suggests that for men, the physical aspects of sex play a much more significant part in arousal than they do for women, for whom ambience, mood, and relaxation are at least as important."

This idea—that sometimes arousal can create desire, rather than the other way around—is also borne out by the research of Rosemarie Basson, a Canadian sex researcher and therapist, who observed that couples in long-term relationships often do not experience as many spontaneous sexual thoughts or fantasies as they used to. Says couples counselor Michele Wiener-Davis in her important book on the subject of mismatched libido, *The Sex-Starved Marriage*: "Being touched in stimulating ways often leads to arousal. Arousal triggers a strong desire to continue being sexual. Hence, desire *follows* arousal."

Sex is both a poison and its own antidote. When couples aren't having sex or the kind of sex they'd like to be having, the silence, anger, and resentment between them is indeed a poison. And sometimes simply having sex, or talking about the sex you'd like to be having, is the antidote.

Love at First Hard-On?

From Romeo and Juliet to *Titanic*'s Leo and Kate, we are drawn to the romantic notion of love at first sight. But is love at first sight a specifically male way of seeing? Are men more likely to experience the phenomenon than women? In my surveys of couples, when asked, "At what point in your relationship did you know for sure that you wanted to spend the rest of your life with each other?" invariably the guys were much more likely to have had definitive feelings at the outset, whereas most women said they needed time to make up their minds.

Indeed, scientists have observed that, when falling in love, there is greater activity in the parts of the male brain associated with visual processing than there is in the female brain. Says anthropologist Helen Fisher, "When the time is right and a man *sees* an attractive woman, he is anatomically equipped to rapidly associate attractive *visual* features with feelings of romantic passion. What an effective courtship device."

So when it comes to sex, do men and women see differently? And does visual stimulation play a much greater role in male sexual excitement than in female arousal?

When the folks at Pfizer conducted their clinical trials of Viagra on men, in conjunction with porn, they came to the unequivocal conclusion that visual stimulation plays a key role in male sexual excitement. When they conducted similar clinical trials with women, the porn did little to spark desire. Is it as simple as concluding that men are visual creatures and women are not? Or is it that women need more than *just* visual stimulation, whereas men often do not? Or maybe women are indeed just as visually oriented as men, but much of the porn is male-centric?

Most of the women I've spoken with say that porn can be a turn-on, but it's not something they'd watch on their own; it's part of the larger experience of being with a *particular* guy. There's even data to support that women are playing a larger and larger role in selecting porn with men. But I surveyed more than a hundred men and women and asked them each, "Have you ever ordered a porn film alone in a hotel?" All of the men had done so (except for those who had never stayed alone in a hotel where porn was offered), but interestingly, only a tiny percentage of women had done so, and more out of curiosity than an interest in being aroused.

But there's a very vocal, and quite possibly correct, camp that insists that women *are* as interested in porn as men, but that porn caters largely to men's interests, consequently alienating women. In the 1980s, Candida Royalle, a pioneer in adult film making, started making porn for women. In her own words, this is what she set out to do with her Femme Fatale Films:

> I created the Femme line to put a woman's voice to adult movies and give men something they could share with the woman in their life. I like to call my Femme movies 'sensually explicit,' or as one viewer described them, the 'Rx for couples.' You'll find them to be less graphic and lacking in the traditional 'money shot,' a staple of most adult films. You'll also find story lines, good original music, and real characters of all ages.

Does her prescription work? Here's what she had to say about a scene from one of her films, *Urban Heat*, that was put to the test in a clinical environment:

> This scene was selected for a study on what actually turns women on. Dr. Ellen Laan showed a group of women a hardcore scene from a typical male-oriented porn movie, and she showed the same group of women the scene . . . from *Urban Heat*, which is considered 'women's erotica.' The women's sexual response was monitored, and afterward they were questioned about how they felt. In a nutshell, women seemed to respond physically to both, but their subjective responses were very different in that they felt shameful and disgusted by the male porn and felt more accepting and positive about their feelings and reactions to my scene from *Urban Heat*. This study was reported in professional journals of sexuality as well as an August 13, 1995, article in the Sunday *New York Times* "Week in Review" section.

Candida Royalle is still going at it. Joining her today is a new generation of porn created by women for women.

The jury's still out on whether women are as visually stimulated by porn as men and if sales of female-centric porn will ever come marginally close to that of their male-centric counterparts. Hopefully it will prove to be a deliberation worth watching.

Follow Your Nose.
It Always Knows.

While men may be more visually oriented than women when it comes to sexual attraction, there's been clear science to support that women have a keener sense of scent than men and that olfactory stimulation plays a much stronger role in female arousal than in men. In short, follow your nose; it always knows.

In one of my surveys of sexual attitudes and behaviors, I asked both men and women to rate various factors in sexual attraction, including features such as eyes, breast size, sense of humor, fashion taste, and so on. In the vast majority of responses I received from women, "his smell" rated extremely high on the list and was often cited amongst the top five factors in sexual attraction, along with confidence, height, a sense of humor, and a handsome face. In men, a woman's scent was consistently rated among the least important factors in sexual attraction.

But that doesn't mean that men don't respond to scent without realizing it. A recent Swedish study concluded that men and women respond differently to two odors that play a role in sexual arousal: a testosterone derivative produced when men sweat and an estrogen derivative found in women. These odors are thought to be pheromones, chemicals emitted by one person that trigger a reaction in another. According to the *New York Times,*

> The estrogen-like compound, though it activated the usual smell-related regions in women, lit up the hypothalamus in men. This is a brain center that governs sexual behavior and, through its control of the pituitary gland lying beneath it, the hormonal state of the body. Interestingly, the testosterone-derivative lit up the hypothalamus in women, but acted as a normal smell in men. The two chemicals seemed to be leading a double-life, playing the role of odor with [the same] sex and of pheromone with [the opposite sex].

If a couple's "odor-prints" don't match, they won't make for a good fit. The source of a person's unique odor, in fact, derives from his/her respective immune system. According to *Psychology Today,*

> A part of our DNA called the major histocompatibility complex (MHC) is involved in producing our own singular smell. Immunity is inherited from both parents, and because the human species is best protected by the broadest array of disease resistance, we are designed to mate with a partner whose MHC profile differs from our own. As such, studies suggest that we like the scent of people with immune systems unlike ours.

To test the theory that the DNA of differing immune systems drives sexual preference, Claus Wedekind, of the University of Bern in Switzerland, conducted a study in which women were asked to smell various clothes worn by different men and select the ones they found sexiest. The women selected the shirts belonging to men whose immune-system profiles most differed from their own. Proving the power of this discovery, many women also said that the favored clothes reminded them of current or ex-lovers. Interestingly, clothes belonging to men who had similar immunity profiles reminded the women of male family members, such as their fathers or brothers. Wedekind writes, "This indicates that MHC-dependent body odor preferences play a role in actual mate choice." So when it comes to mating, it appears that opposites do attract. It's better to pick a partner who is genetically dissimilar, and often the best way to find him is to follow your nose. No wonder that a woman's power of scent is at its strongest during ovulation.

Hard Times Ahead

Dear Ian,

My guy often loses his erection. What's the difference between Viagra, Levitra, and Cialis? Are they basically the same, just with different names, or do they do different things? As a woman, I see all the commercials, but I'd like to know what to potentially expect.

—Amanda, thirty-two, office manager

All of these drugs basically inhibit the enzyme PDE-5, and, therefore, enable muscles in the arteries of the penis to relax and widen. This ultimately encourages blood to flow more easily into the penis to create an erection.

It's no surprise that new competitors to Viagra have popped up, given that as many as 150 million men worldwide potentially experience erectile disorder.

Levitra takes effect more rapidly and supposedly has fewer side effects. Cialis lasts up to thirty-six hours, so couples don't need to feel they have to have sex as soon as he pops a pill. We're only just starting to get clinical data and reports back from doctors about how the competitors stack up against Viagra. Many men like to experiment and find the pill that's right for them. Such explorations must happen under the care of a medical doctor, however, for none of these drugs are without potential side effects.

As of writing this, more than 30 million men have been prescribed the drug worldwide. Annual sales are worth nearly $2 billion, with approximately six prescriptions written per second. And while erectile stimulants have proven a godsend to older men struggling with erectile impairment, as the *New York Times* notes, the pharmaceutical industry makes no bones, as it were, about its intention to enlarge its customer base, contending that erectile disorder is now of epidemic proportion, and that "the face of ED now is a younger, seemingly much healthier guy."

Yet if erectile disorder is, indeed, approaching epidemic rates, shouldn't we look at correlations between the rise in ED and the rise in obesity, stress, and sedentary lifestyles? According to Dr. Irwin Goldstein of the Center for Sexual Medicine at Boston University. "Impotence can be one of the earliest signs that something else is not working."

So, perhaps the flaccid penis is the new icon of the overweight, stressed out, sedentary American man and a condition that shouldn't be medicated away with Viagra, but treated on a holistic level.

Whether a guy actually *needs* an erectile stimulant or not, advertising campaigns for Viagra and its ilk have exploited male anxieties surrounding "ideal" firmness and duration of erections, the very anxieties that often lead to ED in the first place.

Like people, erections don't respond well under pressure. As one *New York Times* reporter noted, "Many men take Viagra to offset the pressure they feel to perform perfectly in a hypersexualized age."

Surely it's the power of this marketing message that emboldens young men in their twenties to say of Viagra, "I like how it makes me feel; it gives me power." But would those men feel as powerful if they knew that the vast majority of nerve endings that contribute to female pleasure are located on the surface of a woman's vulva and that no penetration whatsoever is required for a woman to be stimulated to orgasm? Without his erection or Viagra to stimulate that erection, a man may not feel as sexually virile, but he would possibly prove a more satisfying sexual partner.

As the *New York Times* noted of this Golden Age of the Erection, major pharmaceutical companies have launched multimillion dollar marketing campaigns to redefine erectile dysfunction as a quality-of-life issue for significantly younger men: "The response of the drug makers is, essentially, what's wrong with that?"

Clearly, they aren't asking the thirty million women who will be on the receiving end of those erections. In fact, the media rarely, if ever, alludes to the female perspective on erectile stimulants and how they are reshaping women's intimate lives, altering "sexpectations," and often relegating female pleasure to an afterthought. It's as if all of those commercials depicting happy, contented wives basking in the glow of their husband's newfound potency are being taken at face value and accepted as fact.

Prior to the pharmaceutical treatment of impotence, couples

dealt with the issue through intimacy-building exercises, erotic creativity, and communication. Couples were encouraged to spend more time on desire-building activities, such as communication, foreplay, fantasy, and manual and oral stimulation. Men were encouraged to make love with more than just their penises. The irony is that while these activities didn't always lead to consistent erections, they did often result in greater intimacy, stronger relationships, increased desire, and, yes, more female orgasms.

Before Viagra, men were significantly more likely to address erectile dysfunction holistically. Now, a little blue pill solves the problem. But it does so in a way that's purely physiological, often to the detriment of psychological factors. It's become a lethal part of our culture's sexual shortsightedness and limited romantic attention span, or what I call SADD, sexual attention deficit disorder. As the *Journal of Canadian Family Physicians* recently noted, "Individual psychological, and couple, factors remain important causes. Combining medical treatments with individual, couple or sex therapy is often more helpful than prescribing medicine alone."

Even so, it's virtually unheard of for a medical doctor to recommend a program of sex therapy along with a prescription for an erectile stimulant. And as prescriptions for these drugs become more commonplace, there is far less communication about the condition itself, both within the doctor-patient relationship and the long-term romantic relationship. Instead, we rely on the cultural shorthand embodied in the pill itself, as well as its pervasive branding, to avoid the personal, often difficult, task of communicating about sexual issues and conflicts.

Viagra and its brethren not only reinforce the same old bad habits and often recreate the same old bad sex, but also refocuse the lens more intensely on coital sex, with the penis as its totem. As one woman noted to me about the introduction of Viagra into her sex life, "It's like his penis is a trophy for a game he never played and shame on me if I don't get in there and act like a cheerleader."

With or without Viagra in their lives, many women have resigned themselves to orgasmless relationships and often resort to faking it in lieu of bruising the fragile male ego or prolonging an already uncomfortable or unpleasant activity. And because many of us were taught that intercourse is the "right" way to experience orgasm, many women feel that they are responsible for their nonclimactic state of affairs. With its focus on physiology rather than the holistic sexual landscape, Viagra continues to subordinate female sexuality to a phallocentric model, creating yet another reason for women to feel responsible, unsexy, inadequate, and guilty, rather than fed up and underserved, when their penis-pill-popping partners leave them unsatisfied.

So, if your guy is on an erectile stimulant or thinking about going on one or if you discover some little blue pills in his wallet, I urge you to use this as an opportunity to open up new channels of communication. Remember, regardless of age, a big part of why he's taking an erectile stimulant is because he wants to pleasure you. But, as we discussed earlier, he needs to know that there's more to sex than simply having an erection. And it's your job as a passionista to show him the way.

Plateau

As men cycle through arousal, they reach the plateau phase, which lasts anywhere from thirty seconds to about two minutes. The prostate and testicles swell, the pelvic floor muscles tighten, and men often release a drop of clear fluid. He's fast approaching the point of ejaculatory inevitability, a point in the plateau phase where, with or without further stimulation, he's going to ejaculate. This does not occur with women. Even if a woman is teetering on the brink of climax, she can still lose her orgasm if there's a sudden change in stimulation.

I think that men and women fundamentally misunderstand this important difference in their respective processes of sexual response. On the one hand, women often don't recognize when a man has crossed the threshold of no return; even if there's a change or total cessation of stimulation, he's still going to come. Men, on the other hand, often think that a woman has reached a point of orgasmic inevitability and, therefore, cease clitoral stimulation at the mission-critical moment to enter a full-throttle rush to mutual orgasm, even though the process of sexual response can be interrupted right up to and into climax. In both men and women, the plateau phase is an intense and exciting period. The body and mind are on the brink of total surrender. But it's also a phase that isn't indulged in nearly enough. Men typically crash straight through to ejaculation, and women often get a taste of the orgasmic release to come, only to have it abruptly ceased, deferred, or abridged.

Hot sex is all about recognizing when he's in the plateau phase and keeping him there as long as possible, often bringing him right to the edge of orgasmic inevitability, only to turn him back around.

* * * * * * * * * *

Dear Ian,

Lately, whenever my boyfriend and I have sex, he needs to pull out and finish himself off by masturbating. Is this normal? What's the deal?

—Michelle, twenty-nine

All guys experience a point of ejaculatory inevitability during sex when, with or without further stimulation, they're going to achieve an orgasm. But most guys differ vastly in terms of the amount of stimulation it takes to reach that point: some guys require very little stimulation to reach orgasm; others require significantly more stimulation over a longer duration of time. As guys age, they usually require more stimulation. So is there an age gap between you and your guy? Also, things like condom use, stress, alcohol consumption, and medication can all seriously affect how a guy cycles through the process of arousal and particularly his ability to push through the point of ejaculatory inevitability, which, like the last lap of a race, often requires a final boost of extra energy and concentration. When he pulls out and masturbates, he's basically trying get over the hump.

Next time he pulls out, put your hand over his and use some manual stimulation of your own to "finish him off"—it will help you feel more connected to his orgasm. Also, in between sex sessions, practice your kegels (clenching and unclenching your pubococcygeus [PC] muscles) and then clench them during sex when he's approaching orgasm, which will apply more pressure on his penis.

Also remember that sometimes a little novelty and fresh sensory stimulation can often do the trick. When sex becomes routine, it sometimes becomes harder for a guy to have an orgasm. Sometimes all it takes is whispering something naughty in his ear to give him that little extra push over the edge.

**TOP TEN THINGS YOU ALWAYS WANTED TO KNOW
ABOUT SPERM BUT WERE AFRAID TO ASK***

1. Average volume of a single ejaculation: Around a teaspoon
2. Main Ingredient: Fructose
3. Calories: About 5
4. Protein: 6 milligrams
5. Fat: 0
6. Average speed of expulsion: 25 miles per hour
7. Average duration: 4 to 8 seconds.
8. Average amount of sperm produced over the lifetime of a male: 14 gallons
9. Average number of spurts: 4 to 8
10. Longest money shot in video history: 27.5 inches

*Taken partially from Joseph Cohen's *The Penis Book*.

Orgasm

Put simply, a man's orgasm is the sexual climax that occurs when the penis expels semen in a series of intensely pleasurable contractions. It's simple: *The stronger and greater the number of the contractions, the longer and better the quality of the orgasm.* This is true for both men and women.

What does the male orgasm feel like? I asked a bunch of guys to describe their orgasms, and here's what I got.

"An eruption."
"Pulsating. Throbbing."
"Intense. Quivering."

"Focused in my penis, but spreads throughout my body."

"An explosion, then tingling."

Many studies have shown that male and female orgasms possess more similarities than differences. One study asked both sexes to describe the experience of orgasm and subsequently removed specific references to body parts and gender. The results were then given to a broad team of doctors and psychologists, with the challenge to distinguish which was which. The result? It was even impossible for a group of trained professionals to tell the difference between the men and the women.

A Shot of Happiness

In terms of "ungloved love," studies have suggested that seminal fluid contains beta-endorphins, which can help to diminish feelings of depression in women.

In Jonathan Margolis' *O: The Intimate History of the Orgasm*, he cites the controversial work of Dr. Gordon Gallup at the State University of New York, who maintains that women who had sex without a condom were quantifiably happier than women who had protected sex, based on answers to a questionnaire. Other findings stated that women whose partners did not use condoms became more depressed when their relationships ended; that agitation, irritability, and suicide attempts increased with condom use; and that women with gloved partners took longer to get involved in new sexual relationships than their ungloved-love counterparts. He concluded that some women become chemically dependent on semen. Again, this is highly controversial work, but given that semen contains 60 percent of the USDA recommended daily dose of Vitamin C, perhaps it's only a matter of time before the latest herbal supplement will be sperm-capsules. "Organic," we'll assume.

Shots in the Dark

Regardless of the possible emotional or health benefits, I would not consider engaging in unprotected sex with a partner unless the relationship is monogamous and you have comfortably ascertained that your partner is STI-free.

I probably don't need to tell you that there's no such thing as completely safe sex, but you can, and should, take steps to make sex safer. By using condoms and being careful, straightforward, and smart in your choices, you can significantly reduce the risk of contracting and spreading sexually transmitted infections (STIs).

There are approximately nineteen million new cases of STIs each year in the United States alone, and that number does not account for the large population of people who don't report, or even *know*, they have an STI due to the asymptomatic natures of their illnesses. Also the incidence of STIs is on the rise. It's been estimated that 20 percent of Americans are living with genital herpes and more than 50 percent of women will contract HPV (Human Papillomavirus), which often leads to cervical cancer and infertility. Millions of women are suffering from Chlamydia, which can lead to pelvic inflammatory disease (PID) and infertility. And let us not forget the more than one million Americans living with AIDS and the millions of others who are HIV positive. While many STIs cause lesions, abnormal discharge, or other symptoms, very often they are "silent"—exhibiting no outward signs—detectable only through blood work. For example, we now know that the viral shedding associated with herpes can also occur in the absence of sores. What it all comes down to is the fact that many of us are wholly unaware whether we or our prospective partners are infected with STIs.

Passionistas of the world, take heed! Recent studies show that heterosexual women suffer a higher risk of contracting STIs than their heterosexual male counterparts. For example, the likelihood of transmitting herpes to a partner is approximately 10 percent from an infected woman to a man but 20 percent from an infected man to a woman. It's not fair, but it's true.

Studies reveal that while men are more likely to transmit STIs, women are more prone to ask about sexual history. According to a recent poll conducted by MSNBC and Zogby, 48 percent of the women surveyed claim to check STI status always, compared with only 33 percent of men. This makes it even more crucial for women—who are at a higher risk of contracting a disease—to bring up the subject and know the STI status of their partner(s).

I'm always surprised by the number of smart, educated women who tell me how anxious or embarrassed they feel about introducing the topic of STIs. They're afraid they'll be labeled undesirable or set themselves up for rejection. As one woman told me, "It's so unsexy to talk about your sexual history in the heat of the moment—it's a total killjoy." In addition, many women are concerned that if they insist on the use of a condom, the man will lose interest or his pleasure will be impeded. But caring about your safety should never be regarded as embarrassing, unsexy, or secondary because being comfortable will help you relax and trust your partner and that is the surest route to uninhibited mutual pleasuring and exploration.

Rest assured, if a man doesn't care enough about your safety, comfort, and pleasure to wear a condom, then he's not a smart choice for a partner (or a generous lover, either).

My general rule of thumb is that if you're not comfortable enough to talk to a potential sexual partner about health concerns, than you probably shouldn't be having sex with him in the first place. Good sex requires open communication and honesty. And if you lack that fundamental basis of trust and mutual understanding, chances are the sex is not going to be all that satisfying anyway.

Being educated about sex is more than just accumulating information; it's about having the courage to translate attitude into action. It's about having the confidence in your own desirability to say what you want and need. And let me tell you, *that* is always sexy.

. . . .

Dear Ian,
  I think my boyfriend has been faking it. Is that possible?
      —Eliza, thirty-three, hotel party planner

It most certainly is, especially as more and more guys take selective serotonin reuptake inhibitors (SSRIs) like Zoloft, Paxil, and Prozac. SSRIs boost serotonin levels, which calms us and makes us more even-keeled, but this also has the deleterious effect of inhibiting desire and delaying ejaculation. So if your guy is on an SSRI, it's entirely possible that he's faking it. Encourage him to speak to his doctor if he's suffering from sexual side effects.

It's also possible that your guy is faking it as a function of stress, especially if he's using a condom, which diminishes sensation. Or perhaps he's feeling distant and doesn't want to hurt your feelings. Writes columnist Amy Sohn of an interview with a male faker:

> For men who find themselves starring in their own personal remake of *Endless Love*, he has some advice. "Pump away, give a sudden exclamation of 'Ahh!,' toss your back a bit, and spasm." What if the woman raises suspicions about output? "You say, 'It's not always a lot.' And if you really get down to it, you can say, 'Where's yours?'"

. . . .

Orgasm versus Ejaculation and the Male Multiple Orgasm

With three types of erections, is it any wonder that some experts contend that there are actually four types of orgasm? In her books, sex therapist and former sex surrogate Barbara Keesling maintains that men can experience:

1. A non-ejaculatory orgasm (using the PC muscles or kegels to experience the contractions of orgasm without ejaculation)
2. Multi-ejaculation, in which a man experiences a series of partial ejaculations
3. The aftershock orgasm, in which a guy has one intense orgasm with subsequent less intense aftershock contraction-based orgasms
4. Retrograde ejaculation, or injaculation, in which semen is ejaculated into the bladder rather than out through the

urethra. (Injaculation is mentioned often in tantric sex books as the be-all, end-all of orgasm, while most sex therapists consider it a relatively harmless experience that occasionally occurs.)

While the male multiple orgasm is a great strategy for helping a man get the most out of physical arousal, it shouldn't be confused with female multiple orgasms, which have a genuine basis in physiology. Male multiple orgasms are a technique in which a man experiences the first few pleasurable orgasmic contractions without fully ejaculating. In this sense, it's possible to distinguish orgasm from ejaculation. This is not so with female multiple orgasms, which are genuine. As Natalie Angier wrote in *Woman: An Intimate Geography*:

... the clitoris does not have a venous plexus. In men, this tight-knit group of veins serves as the major conduit through which blood leaves the organ. During arousal, muscles in the shaft of the penis temporarily compress the venous plexus, with the result that blood flows in but then cannot depart, and lo, it is risen. The clitoris does not seem to have a distinct, compressible plexus; the vascularization of the organ is more diffuse. On sexual kindling, arterial flow into the clitoris increases, but the venous outflow is not clamped shut, so the organ does not become a rigid little pole. Why should it? It has no need to go spelunking or intromitting. And it may be that the comparatively subtle nature of its blood trafficking allows the clitoris to distend and relax with ease and speed, giving rise to a woman's blessed gift, the multiple orgasm.

Resolution

Says Jim Pfaus, a psychologist at Concordia University in Canada, to the *Economist:* "The aftermath of lustful sex is similar to the state induced by taking opiates. A heady mix of chemical changes occurs, including increases in the levels of serotonin, oxytocin, vasopressin and endogenous opioids (the body's natural equivalent of heroin). This may serve many functions: to relax the body, induce pleasure and satiety, *and perhaps induce bonding to the very features that one has just experienced with all this.*" In other words, sex isn't just an aspect of love: Sex begets love and is a vital key to its reinforcement.

Bridging the Snuggle Gap

To snuggle or not to snuggle, that is the question. I get complaints all the time from women about guys who don't snuggle after sex, but rather roll over and start snoring.

> HE SAYS: *"After sex, it's like I'm dead. I've been wounded in battle. I need to recover. I need to sleep and heal. I know she wants to cuddle and spoon, but I got nothing left to give."*

> SHE SAYS: *"After sex, I'm tingly and alert. I'm relaxed and happy, but every fiber is alive. If he were up for it, I could definitely keep going. I'm still aroused, and sometimes one orgasm just isn't enough."*

Before you beat up your guy for turning over and snoring, consider that there's a biological basis for why he's shattered and why you're still in a state of semiarousal. Men have to develop the requisite sexual tension to accomplish ejaculation, also known as the propulsive orgasm. It takes a whole lot of blood going into the genitals to accomplish this, and a whole lot of blood flows out after. It's physically exhausting, and prolactin levels go through the roof, giving rise to sleepiness. Since women have no need to ejaculate, blood circulates longer in the genitals: It's slower going in and out. Thus, women remain in the aroused state longer, hence their capacity for multiple orgasms. So if your man rolls over and starts snoring, cut him some slack. Sure, maybe he could use a little retraining (it would be nice if he at least fell asleep *while* holding you in his arms), but his heart may still be in the right place.

A S WE CONTINUE our journey into male sexuality, let us take a page from Joseph Cohen's witty, eclectic volume, *The Penis Book*: "When taking an oath, our biblical ancestors placed their hands over the testicles of a witness to vouchsafe their utmost sincerity and honesty. Words like 'testify' and 'testament' all derive from this unique association."

In the spirit of this ancient tradition, the next time you're unzipping his fly, reach your hand in and make yourself a passionista promise: to strip away the layers of protection and approach his body and mind with a new sense of understanding.

The Male Brain:
The Itch

THE POET W. H. AUDEN wrote that sexual craving is an intolerable neural itch. And true enough, much of our real longing happens in the brain rather than the loins.

· · · · · · · · · ·

Dear Ian,

When my wife and I first met, the sex was so hot and exciting we couldn't keep our hands off of each other. Now it's just not the same. I hate to say it, but sex has become boring.

—Jack, thirty-two, international pilot

Jack's right. We hate to say it, and we hate to hear it even more, because, when it comes to sex, there's no blow more devastating than the sucker punch of "boring."

Boring is the sexual kiss of death. Better to be called freaky, kinky, speedy, rusty, or even crusty (well, maybe not crusty)—or selfish, nervous, erratic, distracted, neurotic, sporadic, uptight, phlegmatic—anything *but* boring.

Yet sexual boredom and lack of interest in sex are probably the two most common complaints I hear from couples, especially, ironically enough, from young ones who are often just a few years into a relationship. In a society that emphasizes instant gratification and quick fixes, the seven-year itch is making people scratch even earlier. And without guidance or a sense of perspective, all of us are too likely to jump ship, or at least jump to the conclusion that our relationship must be fundamentally flawed.

But what if I told you that there was a biological basis for the sexual boredom that often creeps into our relationships? What if I told you that Nature herself ironically stokes the flames of desire, only to douse them later, leaving us with embers that must be reignited to avoid going permanently frigid?

* * * * * * * * * * *

Secrets from the Underground

During my interviews for this book, I asked twenty-five happily married men and women if they would ever commit infidelity in the form of a one-night stand if they knew beyond a shadow of a doubt they'd get away with it, with no consequences whatsoever. Now clearly this wasn't a particularly scientific poll, but of the twenty-five men surveyed, *seventeen* said they'd do it, as opposed to only two women who would.

So what would compel a happily involved guy to take a free pass at a one-night stand?

Remember in my introduction when I said that I'd asked scores of men to describe the best sex they'd ever had? For most of them, it *was with* their current long-term partners. But it was usually at the very beginning of the relationship, when the sparks were flying.

When asked to describe what made the sex so amazing, however, many drew a complete blank. Sure, she may have been enthusiastic in the sack or known her way around a penis, but no, that's not what made it great. What made the sex memorable was the excitement they felt for the other person at the time. And it wasn't limited to a single experience, but rather to the period of time in which the sex was truly amazing, the early days of infatuation.

So I asked this group of men another question: "Is the sex still great?" Here, I received many "yes, buts." *Yes*, they still enjoyed sex (once or twice a week, if even), *but* no, it wasn't nearly as exciting as it used to be. In some cases, the sex had become more affectionate and intimate. But in many instances, it had become flat-out boring. Virtually all of the men surveyed said it wasn't nearly as hot or wild as it was in the beginning of their relationships.

So often did these words, hot and wild, come up, that I felt compelled to ask another question: "In five words or less, describe hot, wild sex."

"Unpredictable, spontaneous. Exciting, new."
"Heart-pounding. Like skydiving."
"Sweaty, dangerous. Going all night."
"Like night driving without headlights."
"Uncontrollable, unstoppable. Totally raw."
"A shot of adrenaline."

Then I asked, "In five words or less, describe the sex you're having now." Here's what the same men said.

"Tender, affectionate."
"Loving. Nice."
"Safe and familiar. Reassuring."
"Consistent. Predictable. Pleasurable."
"Boring. A chore. Same old."

When I asked the guys what had changed about sex over the course of their relationship and why it wasn't still as hot and wild, again, many of them drew a blank. Nothing, they said, had really changed. Perhaps that was the problem.

Sex had become reduced to its rote, physiological components, shorn of its emotional and psychological dimensions, narrowed down to a thin and predictable straight line: beginning, middle, and end. One guy summed it up perfectly.

Sex used to be a jaunt down the yellow brick road: exciting, unpredictable, a Technicolor explosion of sensation and emotion. But now the journey's just not as much fun. Why go to the effort of clicking my heels when I'm already home?

Rarely, if ever, do I hear the complaint of boring sex from couples who have just met or are in the early stages of a relationship. (I do, however, meet plenty of couples who have been together for years and confess that a particular problem in their relationship was always present, but they ignored it, believing it would naturally work itself out.) Sometimes, looking back, couples aren't even sure if the sex was ever really that "hot" because being in love made everything seem so great at the time.

According to *Psychology Today*, one factor that may prove unifying or divisive to a couple is the degree to which their nervous systems are naturally inclined to pursue novel and stimulating experiences. Some of us are natural thrill-seekers, constantly seeking new and exciting stimuli while embracing a sense of risk, marked by a spirit of wanderlust, a love of danger, a hunger for adventure. Others of us are more content with the familiar, reveling in quiet domestic rhythms, intimate rituals (like always celebrating birthdays at the same restaurant), and the joy of knowing someone or something inside out. Nowhere are these differences between "thrill-seekers" and "familiarity-lovers" more apparent than in the area of sexual compatibility.

More than likely, you have some attributes from each of these categories, but you're probably more firmly anchored in one. If you and your partner are both situated at either end of the spectrum, you have the best potential for sustaining a fulfilling sex life together over the long haul. But if you're a sexual thrill-seeker and you're paired with a familiarity-lover, then you will need to work harder to find a happy medium that will simultaneously allow you to get your fix of novel excitement, while enabling your lover to take comfort in familiar routine. Often this differential in your natures will be masked in the beginning of the relationship, when you are awash in the sense of newness. Says Marvin Zuckerman, a psychologist at the University of Delaware, "A person's inherent need for sensation is not necessarily obvious in the early stages of a relationship, when love itself is a novelty and carries its own thrills—it's when the sex becomes routine that problems occur."

Candy Is Dandy

In the early stages of a relationship, our brains bathe us in potent sex chemicals that predispose us to fall in love. We like to say that love intoxicates us, but little do we realize that we really are operating under the influence.

The chemicals that are released during infatuation are the same chemicals triggered when we cheat, which, interestingly enough, are also the same chemicals released when a drug addict gets his or her fix. Says anthropologist Helen Fisher, "Romantic love is an addictive drug. Directly, or indirectly, virtually all 'drugs of abuse' affect a single pathway in the brain."

So what are the euphoric-inducing chemicals that feed great sex and leave us craving more?

As mentioned previously, Ogden Nash wrote that "candy is dandy, but liquor is quicker."

Well, dopamine leaves both in the dust.

In her book, *Why We Love*, Fisher and her team studied the brains of prairie voles, little mice-like critters that, like humans, have a tendency to mate for life. In fact, the prairie vole is among the 3 percent of mammals that remains monogamous. Once they've selected a mate, prairie voles copulate like mad (more than fifty times in two days—*talk about hot and wild*). Then they set about the business of bonding for life: nesting, mating, protecting, and nurturing. In fact, they go through the same stages we do: lust, romantic love, and attachment.

In contrast, the montane vole, a close cousin of the prairie vole, only engages in one-night stands and has no desire for monogamy, despite the fact that they are more than 99 percent genetically similar to their happily married cousins. So what is it about that 1 percent makes them behave so differently? What makes the prairie vole so hot and heavy at the outset, as well as committed for the long haul?

According to Fisher, during that initial frenzy of copulation, dopamine levels in the prairie vole's brain catapult 50 percent, along with significant increases in norepinephrine and oxytocin. The montane vole, however, does not possess receptors for these potent sex chemicals. As the *Economist* writes in an ode to the faithful little prairie vole, "So long as men can keep their hormones potent/They'll be romantic as that model rodent."

In humans, dopamine and norepinephrine are considered natural amphetamines and play a key role in sexual arousal, as well as goal attainment. Dopamine not only helps us focus, but it also contributes to our choice in mates (that harnessing of raw lust into focused romantic love). When scientists reduced the dopamine levels in the brains of female prairie voles, they were no longer faithful or choosy about their sexual partners. In fact, they slutted it up.

No wonder couples in long-distance relationships tend to battle the sexual doldrums better than their cohabiting counterparts: Absence doesn't just make the heart grow fonder, it makes the brain produce higher dopamine levels. Says Helen Fisher, "When a reward is delayed, dopamine-producing cells in the brain increase their work, pumping out more natural stimulants to energize the brain, focus attention and drive the pursuer to strive even harder to acquire a reward: in this case, winning one's sweetheart. *Dopamine, thy name is persistence.*"

But once we're in a committed relationship, sex becomes easier, in a sense, and more readily available. It's no longer a reward, but a given. As one guy commented, "Isn't that the whole point of marriage, so you don't have to worry about not having sex anymore?"

* * * * * * * * * *

Dear Ian,

I'm confused. I've been seeing a guy for the past month, and when I told my best friend that I was holding out and wanted to wait to have sex until I knew it was right, she said, "How quaint." I'm really attracted to him, and it's been hard not to go all the way, so should I just give it up?

—Michelle, thirty-two, pastry chef

My vote is to follow your instincts and enjoy the exquisite torture of delay, which will certainly heighten his sense of anticipation. Today's woman has choices, and you can choose to give it up on the first date or wait it out. I know plenty of happily married couples who slept together on the first date. I also know plenty of women who confuse hooking up with love and wonder why the sex isn't leading to a committed relationship. Regardless of changing sexual attitudes and female sexual empowerment, romantic love is wired into the brain's reward system, and the more a reward is delayed, the more dopamine activity there is. And this natural intoxicator only sweetens the chase. So with that in mind, think of sex as the sublime fruition of hot pursuit and that much more coveted for the delay. Long story short: Every guy loves a good chase, and there's a biological reason why.

* * * * * * * * * *

Love Is a Battlefield

Sometimes the best sex we have is after a heated argument. You may be surprised to learn, however, that the appeal of hot make-up sex has biological underpinnings. Not only does arguing stimulate adrenaline, which produces dopamine, but it's also well known that aggression and orgasm are linked in men. Arguing creates a situation in which love is jeopardized and then (with some luck) rescued with sex. Without a doubt, fighting for some couples is a form of foreplay, which leads to intensely satisfying sex.

"The best part of a fight is making up."

"What can I say? We're passionate people. We fight hard, and we fuck hard."

"The sex is hottest after a fight. We claw and rip into each other with such passion and hunger; it's like we've been starved for each other."

But *must* we fight to love? Some couples have reported that once the fighting diminished, so did the sex. It's as if the two impulses, aggression and eros, drew from the same reservoir of energy. But isn't there an easier way to get the dopamine flowing? Yes. By making like a passionista and getting out on that shaky bridge.

As we progress through a relationship, those sex chemicals that initially drove us wild with passion start to wane. New ones kick in, chemicals that engender a sense of security, well-being, and attachment: vasopressin in men and oxytocin in women. When you are with someone you care about, oxytocin gives you that blissful feeling of completeness when he holds you in his arms. That's one of the reasons it's known as the "cuddle hormone." In men, vasopressin helps him feel protective, and loving and, down the line, paternal.

But sometimes the chemistry of attachment works against desire and romantic love. Helen Fisher observes, "There's evidence to suggest that elevated levels of vasopressin reduce testosterone levels in men." In other words, as men become more attached and more paternal, they often lose desire.

Once those sparks start to wane, we get freaked out and confused. We tell ourselves that our relationships are broken. We feel helpless, rejected. So we cheat. Or we settle into silent recrimination. Or else we cut bait entirely. We don't know how to move forward into the attachment phase while maintaining the excitement of the romantic love phase. Nature pulls the rug out from under us, and we can't seem to find our footing. So we jump on another rug altogether. We are a culture that loves to fall in love but doesn't know how to stay that way. Do we only want what we can't have? Do we prefer the thrill of the chase over the actual attainment of the object of our desire? Is there any way to sustain sexual excitement in a long-term committed relationship? Or are we basically a society of serial monogamists with a fundamental need to refresh our love lives periodically? In short, is there such a thing as a "right person" or "soul mate" with whom we *could* enjoy everlasting passion?

The ancient Greek playwright Aristophanes conjectured that, at the beginning of time, man and woman comprised one creature. Split apart by the gods, we were left to search for our other halves. This search, Aristophanes opined, lies at the very core of love. But is love primarily driven by the desire to *find* our other halves rather than *keep* our relationships whole?

Here's the good news: By understanding the chemistry of desire, we can develop techniques for tricking the brain into stimulating the hot and wild sex chemicals *throughout* a relationship.

In that sense, our brain really is our biggest sex organ. A true alchemist, it has the power to transmute new, raw experience into shimmering desire.

Forget Everything You Ever Learned About Romance

Too often the things we need to emphasize in relationships—trust, familiarity, predictability, and romance—are *not* the building blocks of desire. That's why we need to have a place in our lives that's just for sex: a place that is spontaneous, naughty, bawdy, and unpredictable.

Most of the time, we spend our time making sure our relationship is built on a solid bridge. But if we want to get the dopamine flowing again, we need to have a special place in our lives for sex on that shaky bridge. There's a bit of a sexual thrillseeker in us all, and once the initial thrills of infatuation dissipate, we have to put time and effort into the process of seeking.

Part of the problem for most couples in long-term relationships is that when it comes to sex, we become trapped in the same old, dusty sex scripts that map our behavior from foreplay to goodnight kiss. For most couples, sex becomes a rote, serial process. First comes kissing and hugging. This in turn leads to genital stimulation. That leads to intercourse and orgasm (nearly always his and, hopefully hers). Same ol' thing, same ol' way. And, sure, you may know each other's bodies more intimately and be able to provide each other with more dependable, frequent, even more intense orgasms, but, still, the spontaneity and surprise factors have grown stale.

As therapist Dr. David Schnarch has wisely written of low-desire, sex-starved relationships, "Given the mediocre sex that lies behind common complaints of sexual boredom, low sexual desire often actually reflects good judgment. Rather than focusing on the low-desire partner, clinicians should wonder more about the high-desire partner who often wants more of the usual—often he or she does not know enough about sex or intimacy to realize the sex he or she is having may not be worth wanting."

Whether in or out of the bedroom, couples need to create a sense of novelty. We need to throw away those old scripts and incite a true sense of discovery and surprise. Variety isn't just the spice of life; it's the very life blood of great sex.

The Male Mind:
Overcoming Libido Limbo
and the Fear of Fantasy

FANTASY IS THE engine of desire. Even if a couple's sex life becomes rote or formulaic, fantasy allows us to sheath the familiar in an exciting new skin.

Let me put it another way. From a purely physiological point of view, all orgasms look the same. Blood flows to the genitals (in a process known as vasocongestion), muscular tension (also known as myotonia) builds throughout the body to a peak, and a series of pleasurable pelvic contractions are triggered. That's it—the whole kit and kaboodle.

But surely great sex is more than just maximizing pelvic contractions. As Jonathan Margolis has written in O: *The Intimate History of the Orgasm*,

More than a hundred million acts of sexual intercourse take place every day according to the World Health Organization.

Men and women have practiced procreative sexual intercourse for approximately a hundred thousand years. A back of the envelope calculation suggests, then, allowing for expanding world population since 98,000 BC, that human beings have had sex some 1,200 trillion times.

Fantasy is what makes each and every one of those 1,200 trillion acts of sex absolutely unique. Fantasy is what differentiates us from one another erotically; fantasy confers on us our sexual individuality; fantasy is our sexual fingerprint.

Yet when it comes to sexual fantasy and the male mind, most women don't have the first clue as to what's really going on inside a guy's head. Frankly that's because the flip side of fantasy is fear, and many men are reluctant to acknowledge their inner thoughts to themselves, let alone to a partner. Numerous studies, as well as my own clinical experience, support the fact that many individuals see their sexual fantasies in a somewhat negative light and, thereby, repress them to varying degrees. How many times have I heard a guy say, "If she knew what was going on in my head, she'd think I was some sort of pervert." But the truth is our sexual thoughts and fantasies are so unique that, to anyone else, each and every one of us is something of a pervert.

* * * * * * * * * * *

Dear Ian,

I feel terrible. I frequently find myself fantasizing during sex about men other than my husband. Is that abnormal? I feel so guilty, but I can't help it: Fantasizing helps me enjoy sex, especially after seven years of being together. Sometimes, in the middle of sex, my husband will ask me what I'm thinking about

*(I guess he can tell I'm in another world), and then I lie and say
I'm not thinking about anything. Should I tell him the truth?
Won't he be hurt? I love my husband, but in a weird way, I feel
like I'm cheating on him when I fantasize; so much so that I'm
starting to avoid sex.*

—Ellen, thirty-six, interior decorator

Relax. You're not alone.

Studies have shown, time and again, that people fantasize during sex and not necessarily about the person they're with. Not only is
it normal, but it's also healthy. Sexual fantasy, in and of itself, should
never be construed as a sign that your relationship is in trouble or
that you're dissatisfied with your partner. Quite the contrary, sexual
fantasy is an indicator that you're alive and kicking. As I've said
many times before and will do so countless times again, imagination and sex are consummate bed partners.

Fantasy, a close cousin of dreaming, allows your brain to be
stimulated and entertained, so your body can relax. As neuroscien-
tist Mark Solms, a leading expert in the field of sleep research, ex-
plains, "[D]reaming does for the brain what Saturday-morning
cartoons do for the kids: It keeps them sufficiently entertained so
that the serious players in the household can get needed recovery
time. Without such diversion, the brain would be urging us up and
out into the world to keep it fully engaged."

What this boils down to is that fantasies, much like dreams, free
your brain to explore secret, extraordinary realms without the compunction of practicality, morality, or logic. Flooded by a barrage of
images, memories, and thoughts, your body can basically kick back
and enjoy the show. Fantasy also helps your mind to shut down, an
important component of the female orgasm.

A recent study in which male and female brains were scanned during sexual arousal revealed that women virtually fall into a 'trance' during orgasm and that this brain "deactivity" is necessary for a female to orgasm. A big part of female arousal, much more so than of male arousal, seems to be deep relaxation and a lack of anxiety. Fantasy helps that happen. Says Dr. Gert Holstege of the University of Groningen in the Netherlands, "What this means is that deactivation, letting go of all fear and anxiety, [may] be the most important thing, even necessary, to have an orgasm." So keep fantasizing. Your body and mind are doing what comes naturally for you to experience orgasm. Fantasy allows you to turn off so that you can get turned on.

. . . .

Am I Normal?

The idea that fantasies aren't normal comes from Freud, who declared, "A happy person never fantasizes, only a dissatisfied one." Psychiatrists and the academy jumped on the idea, developing what was commonly referred to as "deficiency theory"—the idea that fantasies signify some deficiency in individuals. A product of the Victorian age, Freud's theories effectively bullied the sexually shamed masses into submission. Today we recognize, even valorize, that sexuality resides on a continuum where normal and abnormal are differentiated by subtle hues of gray.

Sexual fantasy can be a powerful and healthy tool to facilitate intimacy and pleasure. But how we, as individuals, deal with our fantasies—whether we embrace them, repress them, or use them as a substitute for intimacy—will depend on a variety of factors, especially our upbringing. Based on clinical data, approximately one out of four people report some degree of guilt, ambivalence, or fear associated with their sexual fantasies, so much so that it impairs their sex lives.

As an example, individuals from strict, authoritarian, or devoutly religious families are more likely to see their fantasies as forbidden, condemning them as sinful and immoral, based on the view that evil thoughts spawn evil deeds. Some simply find their fantasies embarrassing. Many fear that their fantasies signify mental illness or worry that, unless curbed, thoughts of illicit conduct will eventually bubble to the surface and demand overt enactment.

* * * * * * * * * * *

Dear Ian,

I'm engaged to a great guy. We've been together three years, and we're getting married in two months. The problem is I've started having sexual fantasies about his brother. It started with a sexy dream, but last night I was having sex with my fiancé, and the whole time I was thinking about his brother! Help! The more I try to push the thought away, the more I end up thinking about it. I feel so guilty. Should I call off the wedding?

—Alexandra, thirty-one, computer programmer

First, you have to ask yourself if your fantasies are a legitimate indication of ambivalence about your impending marriage. Is there something going on that you may not be admitting to yourself? The fact that you're fantasizing about your fiancé's brother could be your unconscious way of expressing doubt. It could also be a way of grappling with fears regarding your ability to sustain a long-term relationship through focusing on a taboo with the propensity to destroy your marriage. But if you love your fiancé and feel good about the wedding and your emotional readiness to commit, your fantasy may be nothing more than a "forbidden thought"—it's often the things we're *not* supposed to think about that are the most alluring.

What's more, trying not to think about it is a sure way to escalate the situation and make the thought even more intrusive. In the mid-1980s, a University of Virginia psychologist named Dr. Daniel Wegner, Ph.D., studied the mechanics of thought suppression in an experiment known infamously as the "White Bear Study." Wegner sat people in a room with a tape recorder and told them to say whatever came to mind, with one caveat: No matter what, don't think about a white bear. Yet, no surprise, people mentioned the bear constantly. The more they tried not to think about it, the more they mentioned it. They couldn't stop thinking about the bear, which led the researcher to conclude that by suppressing a forbidden thought, the brain never has an opportunity to process it fully.

So what can we take away from this? Don't let your brother-in-law turn into the white bear. Give yourself permission to enjoy the fantasy, and more likely than not, it will pass. The fact that the fantasy bothers you and feels "out of control" leads me to believe it stems largely from a fear of losing or unconsciously jeopardizing a relationship you cherish, which either statistics or your own past experiences imperil with tenuousness. Ultimately, it's not the fantasy itself that needs to be examined, but your reaction to it and what those feelings of shame, guilt, and lack of control may be telling you. However, if you find yourself growing more and more genuinely attracted to your potential brother-in-law beyond the sexually taboo scenario, you should evaluate the vows you're about to take. After all, sometimes a bear really is a bear, and it may be time for you to get the heck out of forest!

Normal, but Different

So what *do* men really fantasize about? From the racks of porn magazines and advertising eye candy, it would appear, at first look, that big-busted babes enjoy a near monopoly on the male gaze. But it is important to remember that mass media is just that; it's appealing to the broadest common denominator.

The fact that most heterosexual men may be turned on by these images does not mean that this is all, or even foremost, what they individually find erotic. Bluntly put, tits and ass sell. To put it in a more palatable context, if you are an ardent enthusiast of imported chocolate and you're given a Twinkie, you may indulge your sweet tooth. But that doesn't mean that that's what you would want, given a relative choice in the matter. Porn thus exploits a fast-food approach to male fantasy.

The male propensity to objectify body parts stands in marked contrast to women. While certainly appreciative of the male form, most women fantasize about sex within a more emotional, passionate context. In one study of 300 college students, 41 percent of the women but only 16 percent of the men said their fantasies focused on the "personal or emotional characteristics of the partner."

Other salient differences in male and female fantasies are that men are purportedly more likely to imagine themselves taking an aggressive or active role, whereas women often envision something being done to them.

Male fantasies often involve sex with two or more partners at one time. That said, I've observed that while many men fantasize about having a threesome with their partner, the additional partner they're hoping for is not always a woman!

Men also fantasize about being sexually irresistible. They fantasize about their seductive power and ability to overwhelm a reluctant woman through the sheer power of their sexual magnetism. While women are generally the recipients of the male gaze, men, like women, are turned on by being looked at, admired, and desired. Women are often so sadly preoccupied with how they measure up to mainstream standards of feminine beauty and sexual appeal that they fail to recognize that men are likewise insecure about how they hold up to these same oppressive standards. The masochistic upshot of watching pornography for men is that it features men with gargantuan appendages, Herculean endurance, and the kind of cocky arrogance that, in real life, would result in a slap in the face rather than a slap on the tush.

Both sexes enjoy fantasies that center on domination and submission, wielding control and letting go. (What other realm but sex offers such an enticingly open yet private playing ground?) Men are allegedly more likely to fantasize about being aggressors than women, but in my experience, all men have a secret desire to be dominated, and this is one of the keys to understanding and enhancing male pleasure. I'm not necessarily talking about incorporating cuffs and paddles into having sex, but simply allowing a man to experience the act of physical surrender, the alleviation of the pressure to perform, and the license to enjoy sensual and sexual release.

Where do our fantasies come from and how do we liberate ourselves to explore what really makes us tick?

To begin, it's important to understand that there are two basic forms of sexual fantasy: ones that spring from our own imaginations and others that are aroused by external sensory stimuli. Based on my informal surveys, I would say that women are more likely to rely on their own imaginations for erotic fodder (especially during masturbation), while the opposite often holds true for men, who go for prefabricated, visual image-based fantasy. (Women have been fortunate in the sense that they have had no choice but to rely on their own imaginations, while men have been the hapless, easy targets of mass-market masturbatory material.)

Psychologists commonly hold that, for both women and men, internal fantasies are drawn from our unique "love maps," a term first coined in 1980 by Dr. John Money of Johns Hopkins University to describe "the sexual template expressed in every individual's erotic fantasies and practices." In other words, our love maps describe the subconscious blueprint of our erotic desires. The love map lies at the root of our sexual preferences, explaining why we prefer one physical type over another and influencing our sexual fantasies and practices. Each of us has a distinctive love map, as unique as a fingerprint, but there's no real consensus on exactly how our love maps or sexual templates are formed.

Some say early childhood experiences and impressions shape our love maps (beginning with an unconscious tendency to seek out characteristics found in our opposite-sex parents). Fetishes also ostensibly derive from this source, when an early association of an object or image with a sexual stirring becomes emblazoned into our sexual psyches.

Others believe that our early pubescent masturbation fantasies forge our love maps. Early experiences that result in sexual stimulation and orgasm are instinctively repeated.

Is it entirely circumstantial that a teenage boy first masturbates to a typical *Playboy* centerfold and is later drawn to busty blondes? This theory would argue that the image has been imprinted on his love map through the reward of orgasm. It also begs the question of whether the depiction of more realistic, natural women in pornography would result in greater sexual attraction to "real" women than to airbrushed, surgically altered models, thus helping men to escape from the fast-food fantasy fix once and for all.

Still others opine that emotional cravings and unconscious psychological needs inform the love map. An example is the man or woman who gets off on being tied up and bound sometimes simply longs to be hugged and held close. Another is the sexual exhibitionist who had to clamor for parental attention as a child or the voyeur who grew up in a home devoid of intimacy and physical touch. It should come as little surprise that the male desire to be dominated often stems from growing up in a hypergendered household where the pressure to act like a man was ingrained from an early age.

All of these theories have merit, and, in my estimation, there is some truth to each. In the end, our love maps are most likely a dynamic, ever-evolving confluence of factors. Ironically, we often don't know our own love maps, which is why the expression of fantasy, especially via internal triggers that spring from our own imaginations, is all the more crucial: It's our only real way of knowing and sharing our sexual fingerprint.

This is why porn, particularly the ready access of Internet porn, is such a personal bete noire: It's not just the simplistic, erroneous view of female sexuality that bugs me, but the degree to which it creates dependence on external triggers that can both obscure and override the organic development of the love map.

Men deprive themselves of the time to luxuriate in fantasies and desires that are personal and individuated, and they frequently turn to the generic visuals of porn to catalyze the process. More and more men are turning away from their intimate relationships as a source of sexual exploration and settling, instead, for erotic junk food. They often reserve their innermost fantasies for static, air-brushed images and anonymous encounters in chat rooms. Men are more "graphic with their graphics" than they are with their sexually evolved, eager-to-explore partners.

"When I was a kid, I jerked off to magazines, but at least then, I had to fill in the gaps around the pictures. And I remember that as I was masturbating, the girl in the magazine would turn into the girl I had a crush on or, later in life, the woman I was going out with. The photos were a sort of starter. But back then masturbation was an extension of my erotic life. With movies, it became easier. I didn't need to fill in the gaps. Masturbation was less work, and I guess I got lazy. I let the images do all the work instead of using my imagination. But the orgasms also became less meaningful, more disposable. I didn't feel any connection to my own inner erotic life. Now with the Internet, I feel like it's all so . . . external. I don't think I've jerked off inside my own head, without porn of some sort, for years. But it's also lonely and hollow. I always hear that masturbation is healthy, but I wonder if that's true—at least the way I go about it. Masturbation used to be a way of going inside myself. Now it's a way of avoiding life. I used to feel energized and vital after masturbating. Now it just makes me depressed."

—Jonathan, thirty, Web content manager

A S WE APPROACH the end of Part I, it's only apt that you now find yourself at the beginning of navigating the primordial mist of fantasy. Being a passionista means you're ready to explore your own and your partner's unique sexual love maps and figure out all the extraordinary, unpredictable ways the two connect and collide. Through this exciting and dynamic process of self-revelation, exploration, and discovery, you will find your mutual love map, a topography of fantasy and desire particular to you and your partner that can never be duplicated—and trust me, there's enough depth in those waters to support a lifetime of journeys over the shaky bridge.

Bon voyage!

PART

Techniques

TWO

Putting Ideas into Action

L ET"S TALK techniques.

In Part I, we examined male desire and arousal. Now we will look at ways to harness, stimulate, and gratify those desires. We will journey chapter by chapter through the full arc of the male sexual response: desire, arousal, plateau, orgasm, and resolution—and connect thought with action. So, grab your galoshes and buckle your seatbelts because we're in for one hell of a ride.

Before we begin this exciting adventure, here are a few guiding passionista principles from Part I to keep in mind.

1. Like a great literary protagonist, the male pelvis is rife with internal conflict and struggle. A source of epic pleasure and anxiety, it is guarded by layers of protection

at once physical and psychological, conscious and unconscious. As a result, many men are unaware of their extraordinary potential to engage in deeper, more responsive sexual interactions, settling into a narrow set of sex scripts or automated patterns of behavior. Left unchallenged, these protective scripts calcify into mechanistic, static behaviors, which often take the form of male-initiated acts that start with dimmed lights and conclude with intercourse. In other words, it's the same ol' running of the bases we've been doing since high school. To have truly great, *breakthrough* sex, we need to break through all the layers of protection and let go of the tired old sex scripts to create something new.

2. Although the process of male sexual response is laden with nuanced sensations and arousal at every turn, many guys approach orgasm the way a kid does a gourmet dinner— rushing through a spectacular meal to get to dessert. While women are well aware that sex is more than achieving orgasms, for many men, sexual interaction and ejaculation are synonymous. Sex equals orgasm. To help your partner savor the entire meal, you need to help him relax, slow down, and let go, so he doesn't crash through the main course to nab the cherry on the sundae. Remind him. Good things come to those who wait (especially those who say please)!

3. Desire is not merely a light switch that turns on and off with a tug of the genitals. It's the beginning, middle, and end of our sexual encounters and the glue in between. For true desire to flourish, we need to create a sense of hungry anticipation and continue to feed each other's sexual appetites, not just at night in the bedroom, but throughout

our daily lives. After all, why should sex be any more compartmentalized than eating? If we were doomed to ingest the same meal at the same time in the same place until death, chances are we'd get so bored that we'd struggle to consume enough to survive. But we don't approach food that way. We crave and indulge different tastes, different flavors. We eat in different places, at home, on the run, from a quick bite to a Bacchanalian feast. Sometimes we stuff ourselves; other times we have a tasty appetizer and force ourselves to wait until later. Sex should be regarded in the same vein. New flavors, new settings, and new ingredients keep us excited and hungry for more. We don't need a variety of sexual partners to spice up our sex lives; we just need to update the menu more regularly and offer a more inventive selection of daily specials.

4. Sexual excitement is part of the neurology and brain chemistry of romantic love. The stimulation of dopamine is key to our interest in, and pursuit of, sex, as well as our thrill of enjoyment. In the early stages of a relationship, natural sex chemicals fuel our feelings of infatuation. When those chemicals wane, these same glands help generate a chemical cocktail that produces feelings of comfort and attachment. As we move out of the infatuation phase and into the attachment phase, we literally have to trick our brains to "light up again." But it takes more than conventional notions of romance to get the dopamine flowing. We need to find innovative ways to reintroduce elements of surprise, novelty, and mystery to recreate those early feelings of lust. We need to learn how to walk that shaky bridge together.

5. Fantasy is the engine of desire and the lubricant of arousal. Ongoing passion doesn't derive from getting off; it stems from "thinking off." Finding out his fantasies is the key to unlocking his unique turn-ons. While visual triggers like porn have become a quick fix for many a Hungry Jack, they're no substitute for the real thing. Eating on the run may do in a pinch, but eventually all of us crave something more nutritious and filling. While he may be accustomed to the ease of erotic fast food, rest assured that if you take the time to find out his favorite dishes and prepare them with artful imagination, he'll be coming back for more and more.

6. Finally, always remember that great sex isn't about doing something *to* him; it's about experiencing something *with* him. It's about getting to know each other's unique tastes and preferences and exploring new worlds of exotic spices, textures, and flavors. It's the exhilarating, secret journey that you and your partner undertake to reach uncharted realms of passion, pleasure, and intimacy. You're not simply going to play the part of the woman on the shaky bridge; you *are* the woman on the shaky bridge. And you're about to embark on the most exciting adventure of your life with your guy right there by your side.

6

His Sexual Health

WHEN YOU'RE SICK and laid up in bed, very often the first thing to go is the appetite. Sometimes that takes the form of not eating at all, while other times it translates into scarfing down whatever the hell happens to be lying around without regard to taste or nutritional value.

It stands to reason that hunger for sex functions along similar principles. If your guy isn't sexually healthy, he is more likely to skip "meals" altogether or mechanically address his baseline needs in the least exertive, most efficient means possible.

In his book on male sexual health, *The Hardness Factor*, Dr. Steven Lamm cites a British study in which men who reported having three or more orgasms per week experienced a 50 percent reduction in heart attacks and strokes compared to those who had sex less frequently. Lamm's book was inspired by the correlations he made in his own practice between the diminished erectile quality of his male patients and conditions such as obesity, high cholesterol, hypertension, depression, sleep disorders, diabetes, and heart disease: "On the surface, it looks as though the principal message of this study is that having sex reduces the incidence of heart attack and stroke and lets you live longer. In fact, just the opposite is true: *being healthy allows you to have as much sex as you want.*"

So, Is Your Guy Sexually Fit?

Ask a woman if she is sexually fit, and she will tell you straight away to what extent the state of her body impacts and impairs her sexual state of mind. Fat, skinny, fatigued, out of shape, dehydrated, you name it: Women know and understand all *too* well how their sense of physical well-being influences their level of desire. For men, however, much of this is virgin territory. While today, more than ever, men worry about their weight and fitness, their focus tends to be more superficial. If it looks okay on the outside, they're good to go. And because most men tend to have sex with their penises instead of their whole bodies and minds, they often measure their sexual health by the inch, i.e., by how well they can get it up, keep it up, and get it off, even if it requires a little porn or a pill to make that happen. But to have truly embodied and ultimately out-of-body sex, a man has to become more attuned to his entire body, head to head and nape to toe.

So before you embark on your lifelong sexual journey, here are some questions to consider regarding his fitness for long-term travel.

Does he exercise? Regular aerobic workouts keep the blood flowing and the arteries producing nitric oxide. Nitric oxide is the life blood (literally) of the male erection and is essential to sexual arousal. To that end, you'd be amazed how many guys tell me that they often feel their horniest post-exercise. Says Steve, a real estate broker in New York City, "Running the Central Park reservoir is like foreplay for me. Pushing myself physically gets me juiced up, and then I want to channel all that energy into sex. It's like the workout before the workout." Says Peter, a psychologist in Tulsa, Oklahoma, "I feel at my most alive when I'm pushing myself physically during a workout, and, consequently, I feel at my most alive sexually when I make love right after a workout."

These observations aren't surprising: Not only is overall vascularity heightened during aerobic exercise, but also feel-good endorphins that contribute to sexual arousal are released. So next time he heads off to the gym, tell him to wait on the shower until he gets home. Then you can really get his heart pumping with some steamy shower sex!

Exercise also plays a major role in generating positive self-esteem, perhaps the most powerful sexual enhancer. Women aren't the only ones to suffer from diminished desire due to insecurity about fitness and physical appearance. You wouldn't believe how many men suffer from poor body image. And as women know all too well, low self-esteem dampens sexual desire.

On a personal note, I was way over my ideal weight not too long ago, and I was basically stuck in a low-level sex rut (being an anxious, sleep-deprived father didn't help, I should add). I rarely exercised. Not only did I not have the energy for sex, but also I just felt downright unattractive. I definitely didn't feel comfortable in my own skin or being seen in the buff, for that matter. Then my wife started taking exercise classes, and I made a decision to get in better shape myself. I wasn't going to be left behind. So I went on an exercise and fitness program. Not only did I lose the weight fairly quickly, but also the smallest improvements along the way boosted my self-esteem and libido tenfold. It wasn't about getting the perfect body or looking like a Calvin Klein model, but about getting myself to a place where I was more energetic and confident. I went from a lights-off to a lights-on attitude and from being sexually stagnant to sexually charged. It wasn't about my attraction to my wife (which was never in doubt), but rather my sense of *being* attractive, both *to* my wife and in general. So what's the lesson? Not only are both exercise and diet vital to sexual vitality, but also, for both men and women, when weight is up, body image and libido go down (and for men, down is never good).

Is he eating well? A poor diet is a major contributor to heart disease, high cholesterol, arterial plaque, and high blood pressure, among other conditions, all of which inhibit blood flow to the penis and negatively impact erectile quality and desire. So what's the desire-diet key? Eat for the heart, and you're eating for desire. Now I'm not about to prescribe a precise food regimen (there are enough diet choices on the bookshelves without adding another to the mix), but I will tell you that when the ratio of nutrients to calories in a food is high, as is the case with most vegetables, fat burns off, and health is maximized. Hence, the more nutrient-dense foods you consume, the more you will be satisfied with less calories, and the less you will crave more high-calorie foods. So don't eat to live—eat to love, too!

Is he stressed out? Not only does stress mar sexual performance, but the medications commonly used to treat it, such as antianxiety drugs, tend to depress the libido and inhibit desire. But with or without pharmaceutical aids, men, like women, feel less sexual when they're emotionally distressed.

· · · · · · · · · · ·

Dear Ian,

My husband and I have never before had a problem with sex (we've only been married for two years, so I guess we were still in the honeymoon stage—at least up until recently). But in the last couple of months, things have taken a turn for the worse, and we're stuck in a rut. My husband didn't get a promotion he was counting on, and now he says he wants to wait before we try to have a baby, which has crushed me. We just seem to be angry at each other all the time. In bed, it's like I'm lying next to a stranger. I've never felt more alone.

—Debbie, twenty-nine, public relations manager

Well, Debbie, you're certainly not alone. While financial issues are the number one cited reason for divorce in the United States, sexual issues are a close second (and it is safe to assume that sexual dissatisfaction is highly underreported). But, the truth is the two are insidiously intertwined: Financial stress often facilitates and intensifies sexual discontent.

In my practice, I've found that one of the main reasons for loss of libido in men is financial worries. And in your situation, the pressure to have a baby "on schedule" is compounding this anxiety. Take these two factors—loss of an anticipated promotion and pressure to procreate—and you begin to understand why he's avoiding physical intimacy. But not having sex only makes matters worse, exacerbating your respective isolation and eroding the foundation of your marriage.

Men often suffer silently through problems or lash out irrationally, rather than engage in constructive communication. Right now, he perceives you and your wants as part of the problem. You need to show him that you're part of the solution instead.

Just because he says he wants to put off trying to have a baby doesn't mean he doesn't want one. Far more likely, he is not only disappointed, but he also feels guilty and possibly even emasculated about having to delay your family plans. While women often believe that there will never be a perfect time to have a child, one of the main reasons why men put off fatherhood is that they don't feel ready. This sense of readiness is often intrinsically connected to a sense of financial confidence.

In the short-term, you need to let go of your pregnancy timetable, take some pressure off, and reestablish your bond as a couple and a team. Not only will a return to sex for pleasure reinvigorate your relationship, but it will also revitalize his approach to life and help confer on him the confidence and sense of assurance he needs to meet and overcome his other life challenges. It will remind him that you value him for who he is rather than for what he can provide you.

You'll find that the love you give will soon be surpassed by the love you receive (and, eventually, conceive).

* * * * * * * * * * *

Is he sleeping well? As vital to our physical well-being as food and water, a good night's rest often finds its expression in his morning erection. So don't hesitate to give him a routine morning exam.

Is he taking his vitamins? L-arginine, an amino acid, is a building block of protein and converts to nitric oxide, which, as we discussed earlier, is vital to sexual arousal. Pycnogenol is a combination of many antioxidants extracted from the bark of a pine tree and is known to protect the heart, fight those nasty free radicals, and increase sexual arousal. Omega-3s, which are found in certain fish, also reduce plaque that builds up in arterial walls and impairs blood flow. Vitamins C and E are powerful antioxidant supplements that protect against free radicals and reduce fatty deposits in the blood. Most of these vitamins and minerals will be found in a quality multivitamin.

With a combination of a balanced diet, exercise, stress management, and some good old-fashioned erotic creativity (more of that to come), your guy's going to be fit as a fiddle and living his love life to the fullest.

Turning Foreplay into Moreplay

ONE OF THE cardinal rules of writing (post-high school) is never introduce a topic with a dictionary definition. Yet when it comes to foreplay, so many of us are leading dictionary-definition sex lives that I've decided to break the rule.

Main entry: foreplay
Pronunciation: fôr-"plA
Function: *noun*
1: sexual stimulation preceding intercourse
2: action or behavior that precedes an event

If you've read Part I, my problem with this definition will come as no surprise: It positions intercourse as the main event and implicitly diminishes everything that comes before (and after).

With its emphasis on sexual "readiness," foreplay, as defined and practiced, focuses more on stimulating physical arousal than sparking desire. If you'll recall, a little earlier we spoke of the three distinct types of male erections: psychogenic (or mentally inspired erections), reflex erections (that occur as a result of direct genital stimulation), and nocturnal erections (that occur spontaneously). Our basic societal conception of foreplay endorses the reflex-based approach to sexual interaction, at the expense of a truly impulse-based psychogenic approach. As a result, we often struggle to create desire from physical arousal, cajoling the brain to follow the body when it should be the other way around.

· · · · · · · · · ·

Dear Ian,

My boyfriend and I are living together, and we're both really focused on our jobs at this point in our lives. We haven't had time for sex, or much else for that matter, for several months. We've tried to schedule sex, but it's just not working. My boyfriend says that where there's a will there's a way, but the problem is that we've made time for the way, but I just don't have the will anymore.

—Rebecca, twenty-six, C.P.A.

For couples leading hectic professional lives, scheduled sex has become fairly commonplace. Unfortunately, structuring sex into a weekly schedule only compounds performance pressures and undermines spontaneous desire, reducing sex to another task that must be squeezed into the to-do list, much like taking multivitamins or doing sit-ups.

No wonder the scheduled sessions aren't working: You're halfheartedly going through the motions, relying on a mechanical sense of arousal to get you going rather than a genuine desire to pleasure each other and connect intimately. In a healthy, long-term relationship, desire isn't about fulfilling a general need to have sex, *but rather desiring sex with a particular person.*

Another downside of scheduled sex is that it rarely meets our expectations for intimacy and often reinforces the very sense of disconnectedness we're trying to overcome. I'm not saying that showing up isn't half the battle, but if that's all you're doing, then you're missing out on the other half.

So why don't you keep your one-on-one sessions on the calendar as an opportunity to spend quality time together, but remove the pressure to have sex? If you do have sex, fine, but if not, don't sweat it.

Also, why not think about taking a personal day or calling in sick together, and then go out and "play hooky" as a couple: Sleep in, take a long walk, a luxurious lunch, hold hands, go to the movies, and just *enjoy* each other's company. An hour or so a weekend after an exhausting and stressful week of work is hardly enough time to relax, let alone recharge your relationship batteries. My guess is that if you spend more unstructured, pressure-free time together you will find you have more time in your busy schedules for pleasuring each other than you think.

* * * * * * * * * * * *

When it comes to foreplay, it's time to stop confusing arousal with desire. Foreplay is not a few mechanical strokes or flicks of the tongue that give rise to an erection and lubrication. Foreplay is the mental component of sex. *Foreplay happens outside the bedroom;* I'll say it again: *Foreplay happens outside the bedroom* (or wherever else you'll be pleasuring each other). All of that scrumptious kissing, touching, stripping down, nibbling, teasing, and sucking—that's not foreplay: It's *coreplay.*

I'm not saying that foreplay can't, or shouldn't, include physical interaction (in fact, we need much more physical intimacy in our lives outside the bedroom), but it's important to break out of the physical reflex-based approach. It's time to let the brain lead and inspire the body to follow.

By no means does foreplay always need to lead to intercourse or even orgasm. Remember back in high school when the possibility of a quick kiss or a stolen smooch with your sweetheart was enough to make you sneak out a window past curfew? That's the feeling we're talking about.

Think of great sex as a favorite novel: Every word, every page, and every chapter adds up to the whole. The pleasure is in the experience of reading rather than finishing the book, the enticement of "opening" something new because of the excitement of never knowing what you will discover "between the covers."

SEXUAL DESIRE SHOULD similarly stand above and beyond any single act of sex. Sometimes a sexual interaction is a mere phrase, sometimes a chapter, sometimes a full book you read over and over before moving onto the next, keeping its memory alive in your thoughts, transforming you, if just a little, forever. On a simpler level, studies have shown that intermittent rewards are more powerful than consistent rewards. Being erotically charged by your partner does not mean that every interaction has to end with sexual gratification.

I often talk about being erotically engaged with life, and I don't mean suddenly transforming into a nymphomaniac. The term "erotic" is derived from *eros*, which is the Greek word for romantic or sexual love. But Freud had a different definition of eros. He said that eros is "the life instinct innate in all humans."

On this point, the vaunted cigared-one and I couldn't agree more. Eros isn't just about sexual lust; it's about a lust for life. And foreplay is not about sex. It's about infusing our relationship with a sense of eros.

. . . .

Dear Ian,

How can I talk to my boyfriend about sex stuff without him flipping out and going postal on me?

—Elizabeth, twenty-three

Trust me, you're not alone. Just recently a female patient of mine recounted the harrowing experience of trying to talk to her boyfriend about his lovemaking skills. "It was like a scene out of *Taxi Driver*. He gave me this Robert De Niro *'you talking to me'* look, and then pointed his finger in my face. I swear I thought he was going to off me!"

When it comes to communicating about sex, there's often a gap between what we want to say and how we end up saying it, and even the gentlest of words can come off as confrontational. Criticism, expressed or perceived harshly, is the sexual kiss of death.

Anthropologists have long observed that women are "face-to-face" communicators, while men do so "side-by side." This means that women are much more comfortable with direct eye contact, which probably has a lot to do with the female history of nursing, cuddling, and generally fawning over their infants all the while staring lovingly into those big baby eyes.

Men, on the other hand, find direct eye contact extremely confrontational. As Helen Fisher wrote in her remarkable book, *Why We Love*, "this response probably stems from men's ancestry. For many millennia men faced their enemies; they sat or walked side by side as they hunted game with their friends." So unless you want your words to send him into battle, use evolution to your advantage and have a sex talk with him while taking a walk or drive, or just sitting comfortably next to each other on the couch.

Prepare yourself: Take the time to really think through what you want to say, with as few generalities as possible. When it comes to sex, men need specifics. It's not enough to just say you want more foreplay or less routine; you need to think of one or two "time and place" examples of when and how things could have been different.

Solve your own problem: Have a "sexy solution" in mind. Maybe the answer is more oral sex, more cuddling, or more fantasizing. No matter what issue you'd like to discuss, think about the ideal solution and how to present that solution in a sexy, constructive way.

Making the Leap

OURS IS AN EXTREME CULTURE. From extreme sports and extreme makeovers to the extreme ways in which we work and play (even our favorite reality TV shows are growing more extreme by the season), we thrive on the intense rush that comes from taking risks and pushing ourselves to our physical and emotional limits. So then if adrenaline and endorphins are our bodies' natural drugs of choice, isn't it time we consider taking on a little extreme sex?

If you think I'm talking about having sex while going skydiving, well, you're right; I mean sort of.

Sometimes, in my clinical practice, I like to do a fun exercise with couples to get them thinking and talking—often for the first time—about what really turns them on.

I start by showing them an unedited DVD of real people

skydiving for the first time, complete with screaming, cursing, and even hysterical crying that's typical of that primal jump, as well as the whoops, hollers, and howls of joyous exhilaration that follow.

Next, I ask each of them to take a moment and think about one thing that really gets him or her sexually excited. It could be a fantasy or a particular sex act, even a strange position they always wanted to try, but it has to be some secret thing they've never shared with anyone else before.

Then I ask them to phrase their sex thought as an "I want" statement (for instance, "I want you to do me up against the wall in the basement stairwell"), but not to utter that statement aloud . . . *yet.*

Next, I place a narrow one-foot bench in the center of my office, and I ask the couple to hold hands and step up onto it together.

Then I say, "Close your eyes. Imagine you're on a plane, flying thousands of feet above ground, perched by the cabin door, about to parachute down through the great blue beyond together. Now, instead of jumping off the bench, when I say *go* I want you to shout out your 'I want' sex statements at the same time."

Now some of you may be thinking I'm taking this whole skydiving metaphor a little too far (or perhaps not far enough for some of you true extremists). But, the truth is, for *most* of us, the very act of revealing our secret sexual selves to an intimate partner is as daunting and terrifying as jumping out of a soaring plane, if not more.

Many of the exercises I do with couples involve stepping, slowly but surely, outside their sexual comfort zones. This is what I call taking "safe risks." Time and again I have seen that even the smallest, "safest" risk will reward a couple with the sense of newness and novelty that is crucial to dopamine production and sexual excitement. It helps foster an attitude toward sex that is inquisitive, adventurous, bold, and empowering.

In no particular order, here's a list of what some of the guys have shouted in their "I want" sex-jump statements.

"I want to spank you."
"I want to tie you up."
"I want you to tie me up."
"I want to watch you touch yourself."
"I want to role play."
"I want to have sex with the lights on."
"I want to have sex in public."
"I want you to go down on me more often."
"I want to have a threesome."
"I want you to wear sexy lingerie."
"I want to make you come with my tongue."
"I want [you] to shave your genitals."
"I want to have anal sex."
"I want to watch you get it on with another girl or guy."
"I want [you] to talk dirty."
"I want to take naked photos of you."
"I want to make a sex video."
"I want us to watch porn together."

A list of women's "I want" statements have ranged from requests for more oral sex to a wish to dominate or be dominated. In fact, the couples are frequently startled to discover that their secret innermost desires aren't so different.

After the couple makes their jump statements, I repeat each of their statements aloud just so there's no confusion. Then, I ask them to clasp their hands together and step down from the stool: One small step for woman- and mankind, one *giant* leap for their sex life.

Now, we begin to discuss what these statements and desires actually mean to and for each other. We talk about how they can continue to experience the exhilarating freefall sexual journey they've initiated in my office in their daily lives, whether through fantasy or action.

What are your jump statements? How do they make you feel? Are they consistent with your values and sense of self, or do they run counter to your social identity? Are you prepared to utter them to your partner and potentially pursue them? Are you ready to hear what your partner has to say and embrace his desires with a positive attitude?

If you're still not entirely sure, then from this moment on, I want you to think of yourself as a white tigress. That's right; you heard me—a white tigress.

Allow me to explain.

Dragon Tails

THE WHITE TIGRESS is the Chinese term for a woman who practices disciplined sexual practices for the purpose of fostering her own health, youthfulness, and rejuvenation. The sexual principles of the White Tigress were developed in ancient China by a secret society of female Taoist sexual warriors and have been scantily documented in Western culture. Think of the passionista as a direct descendant.

Taoist author and historian Hsi Lai was given the opportunity to observe one of the last remaining White Tigresses and learn many of the secret practices with the intention of communicating her wisdom to Western women. He writes in his book *The Sexual Teachings of the White Tigress: Secrets of the Female Taoist Masters*, "A White Tigress may appear and function in any walk of life. She is not restricted by either her social environment or religious beliefs."

While some of the principles of the White Tigress run counter to modern Western thinking, such as the idea that absorption of male sperm by a woman (mainly through oral sex and contact with the skin) can lead to physical rejuvenation and spiritual immortality, the general approach to sex is empowered and emboldened.

White Tigresses were trained in "Absorption of the Male Sexual Energy," also known as "the Dragon's Breath":

> The orgasm emits sexual energy from the body, not only in fluids, but as a substantive psychological force. The Tigress discovers how to absorb and make full-positive use of the fluids and energies of her own orgasm and the male's orgasm to benefit her health and well-being. Absorption is the ability to mentally and physically induce the energy of the orgasm into herself, whereby she then uses that masculine energy to both fortify and enhance her own feminine energy.

White Tigresses traditionally maintained sexual relationships with two categories of men, Green Dragons and Jade Dragons. The former were men who were seduced by a White Tigress purely for their semen and sexual energy. Learn to treat your guy as your Green Dragon. Use him for the pleasure he gives you. Use him for your own sexual contentment. Trust me; he won't mind. Your willingness to initiate and your boldness in taking and making him your personal sex toy will drive him to new levels of ecstasy. He won't know what hit him, and you don't have to tell him. Remember, the White Tigresses were a secretive bunch, and you can keep your new identity to yourself.

The latter category of male consort, the Jade Dragon, was an equal partner to the White Tigress in sexual practices. Their sexual relationship was mutually beneficial.

So I'm telling you now to think about your guy as the Jade Dragon, too. Your willingness to give and take, to initiate and receive, to communicate, express, learn, and share, will make for a sexual relationship that never stops growing, never stops venturing into unexplored avenues of secret pleasures.

As a modern White Tigress—a passionista—you must learn how to find the Green Dragon and Jade Dragon in the same guy, from moment to moment and moon to moon, depending on your ever-evolving individual and mutual desires.

At the heart of the teachings of the White Tigress, however, is a willingness to make sex a critical and essential component of your life. It is allotting plenty of time and a revered place in your busy, hectic lives solely for exploring and experiencing sexual pleasure together. It's making a conscious decision not to relegate sex to a quickie on Wednesday nights and a romp on Saturday afternoons before dinner. It is according your sexual relationship with your partner the vital importance it deserves as the life blood of emotional intimacy.

But before you can do as a White Tigress, you have to start thinking and acting like one.

To a Tigress, a man pushing his penis in and out of her vagina to orgasm is not sex. To her, sex means recreating [youthful] feelings of adventure, romance and playfulness. . . . Briefly said, she seeks the excitement of sex.

When it comes to sex with a monogamous partner, it's too easy to sink into our adult mind-sets and routines, where we are no longer open to learning or experiencing anew. We become focused on our emotional needs, using sex to express those needs, to gauge our compatibility and desirability, instead of allowing sex to release us from the daily rigors of adult concerns, fears, and obligations. In her practice, the Tigress allows for periods of engaging in mild exhibitionism, periods for flirting and showing off to acquire men, and periods for secret sexual interludes. She does all this, obviously, within the context of being an adult, but she attempts to be child-like in her energy and actions.

So go ahead and jump into new and secret worlds of sexual exploration. Give yourself permission to make the leap. Learn to listen without judging and take chances. Let yourself be the subject of desire and have the confidence to know that you can give through taking, without gauging yourself through a man's eyes or erection.

Speaking of erections, the ancient Taoist texts have a saying about the male member: "When the Tigress plays, the dragon whips its tail."

So get playing.

The Passionista Files:
An Oral History

I WANT YOU to close your eyes for a moment and think back to the tumultuous days of youth when sex was still naughty—fraught with mystery, peril, excitement, danger, intensity, and above all else, newness. I want you to dig into the recesses of your memory and rediscover the inimitable joys of pleasuring and being pleasured. I want you to recall the indescribable sense of surprise, exhilaration, and passion that first time you felt, heard, smelled, watched, tasted a lover gripped in the throes of orgasm; the first time you yielded to the power of another person's touch.

These Pleasures That We Lightly Call Physical

The French novelist Colette understood that by labeling our erotic lives as essentially physical, we greatly underestimate the significance of other forces—from psychological to aesthetic—that influence and define our desires and liberate sex from the generic sphere, to give it lasting meaning. By exploring fantasies with our partners—sometimes through words, sometimes through actions—we make our erotic lives dynamic, unpredictable, as forever evolving as we are, creating an endless spectrum of possibilities for mutual discovery, pleasure, and intimacy. So, in homage to Colette's poetic justice,

We sample here what may await; Passionista and her mate.

I Had a Dream

Says Jenny, a thirty-two-year-old investment banker: "I have a very creative sex life, and I owe it all to Dr. Martin Luther King Jr. No kidding. I used to get really nervous talking about sex and fantasies with my boyfriend, Bill, and he's also really shy about that sort of stuff. So we never said much of anything. We're basically sexual introverts, but there was so much I wanted to explore with him, and I knew we weren't fulfilling our sexual potential.

"Then one day I was home from work for Martin Luther King Day, and I heard part of his famous historic speech on television;

that whole 'I have a dream' mantra really stuck with me. The next morning I turned to Bill and said shyly, 'I had a dream.' He wasn't really listening to me, so I said it again: 'I had a dream—a sexy dream.' That's when Bill got curious and said, 'Oh, yeah?' and I made up this fantasy about watching him have sex with another woman.

"At first I was nervous describing it to him, but because I was supposedly 'recounting a dream,' it was easier than I thought it would be. I mean we're not responsible for our dreams, right, at least not consciously? Anyway, it really turned us both on, and he couldn't stop asking me about it. He even called me several times from work, and I let myself get more and more explicit.

"Of course it was only a matter of time before he asked if watching him get it on with another woman was something I *actually* wanted to try. I thought about it for a moment. Then I said no; it was just a sexy dream that I wanted to share with him. And we left it at that.

"But sometimes there are sexual things I *do* want to try and my 'sexy dreams' have become our way of breaking the ice. And Bill has suddenly begun having 'sexy dreams' of his own."

Says Ian: Jenny's "I had a dream" approach to sharing a sexy fantasy is brilliant because it gives her the freedom to express her secret desires and fantasies without feeling judged. Even when Jenny and Bill don't act on the dreams, which is most of the time, Jenny and Bill love to talk about them before and during an encounter: And that invariably leads to great sex. Jenny's habit of sharing her sexy dreams in the morning gives them something to think about all day and creates a strong sense of sexual anticipation.

On those occasions when there is something new that Jenny wants to try with Bill, her "dreams" are a great way of getting the ball rolling. For example, Jenny was interested in trying anal sex for the first time, but she wasn't sure if Bill shared her curiosity, so she made up a sexy dream about it. When Bill asked her if that was something she may want to try, she said it was. And they went on to explore it together.

Jenny has definitely noticed a change in Bill's libido, and his newfound sense of desire is no doubt tied to his increased sense of excitement for Jenny in general. Through sharing her dreams, Jenny has become unpredictable, bold, adventurous, desirous, and even a little dangerous. In short, Jenny has become the woman, maybe even the Tigress, on the shaky bridge.

The "I had a sexy dream" technique is also a great way to initiate a dialogue about a sexual issue that may be troubling a relationship. As an example, one woman I counseled was frustrated by her husband's less than stellar oral sex techniques. Like many men, he was too rough and impatient. She didn't know how to raise the subject without hurting his feelings or making him defensive, so I suggested she express her desire for change as a positive fantasy. She told her husband that she had a sexy dream that he kissed her tenderly all over her body and then slowly teased her to orgasm with his mouth. He didn't even need to ask if that was something she wanted to try. He just did it. And it was a happy ending, indeed.

All the World's a Stage

"In a car, at a bar, in a store, by the door"—sounds like the makings of a Dr. Seuss story. And with a little bit of imagination, there's no end to all the fun places we can play our naughty games.

Let me put it simply: For most guys, a little playful exhibitionism—being sexual in public, or semi-public where there's a risk of being caught or observed—is like a jolt of sexual adrenaline. Not to be confused with public sex, which could get you arrested or at least seriously embarrassed, playful exhibitionism is about making the most of quick moments to stimulate the mind and get the heart pounding. Following are some noteworthy public moments that later, in private, led to momentous sex.

In a dressing room Says Jeff, twenty-nine: "I used to hate going shopping, until I met Tammy. She turns every dressing room into our own personal peep show. She's definitely an exhibitionist. She goes in to try something on, and then she calls me to come in and help her. Sometimes the dressing room has a door, but sometimes it's just a thin curtain that barely shuts all the way. And Tammy likes to go shopping on weekends, when there's always a crowd of people waiting. So she calls me in, and she's usually half-dressed or just in her panties and bra, or in the middle of taking something off. (One time she was totally naked, and I'm sure people could see in.) But she doesn't care, it just makes her bolder, and it totally gets me juiced. Sometimes she makes a play for my pants, but I don't let her. I love the feeling that she just can't wait to get me into bed with her. It drives us both so wild that we usually wind up hopping in a cab to rush home and get it on."

In a restaurant Says Sharon, thirty-six: "Peter's an SVP of sales for a technology company, so we go out to a lot of restaurants with his clients and their wives. I used to get bored and annoyed during those dinners. But then I found a way to keep it more interesting and pick up the pace. I like to put my hand on Peter's crotch under the table and give his cock a firm squeeze. Then I whisper something *really* filthy in his ear about what I'm going to do to him when we get home. A couple of times, I told him I had to go rub myself in the bathroom to relieve some of the tension. Then I came back and surreptitiously brushed my fingers over his lips, so he could taste and smell my need. That definitely got the meal moving faster."

For his friends Says Chloe, twenty-six: "Jake's always having 'the guys' over for Sunday afternoon football, and I like to wear something casual, but sexy, whenever they're here—like a tank top and a pair of cut-off jeans. His friends are always checking me out, and I know it turns him on to know that his friends think I'm hot. I always make sure to kiss him and hang all over him. And I think it gives him a sense of power to be wanted like that in front of all his buddies."

In a taxi Says Sara, thirty-one: "Come on, is there *anything* better in the whole world than fooling around in the backseat of a cab on the way home? There's something about the eyes of the cab driver in the rearview mirror that's a real turn-on. I love to kiss and snuggle in cabs or unzip my boyfriend's fly and put my hands down his pants. Sometimes I'll pull my skirt up high above my legs and close my eyes and let him touch me. One time I took my panties off in the bathroom before getting into the cab and handed them to Jake. It made him crazy. I know the cabbie was probably getting an eyeful, but hey, isn't that one of the perks of the job?"

In nothing but a coat Says Leslie, thirty-four: "Last year I bought this old fur coat and felt hat at a vintage store in the East Village.

Whenever I wear them, I feel like a flapper from the 1920s—I want to go dancing on tabletops. The coat falls just below my knees, and it makes me feel sexy and wild, which is saying a lot, since ordinarily I am self-conscious about my body. I'm the kind of person that likes to have sex with the lights off, or at least I used to be. So, one night my boyfriend and I went to do some midnight shopping at the supermarket, and, without telling him, I wore *nothing* but the coat and the hat. And pointy pumps of course. When I suddenly flashed him halfway down the cereal aisle, he was totally shocked and turned on. Then, as I was pushing the cart down the aisle, I kept lifting the coat to show him a little bit of this and that, and he couldn't keep his hands off me. We went home and had sex on the floor, with the lights on, and I never took off the coat. It was definitely the best sex we'd ever had . . . until I found this red-hooded rain slicker and yellow galoshes at a second-hand store a few weeks later."

With the blinds up Says Ken, forty-two: "We live in brownstone that overlooks a courtyard; it's straight out of Hitchcock's *Rear Window*, with a view into everyone's apartments. Sometimes Candace walks around naked after getting out of the shower, and I know people can see right into our bedroom. I always tell her people are watching, but instead of shutting the blinds, she shrugs it off and says she doesn't care. Once, she pushed me onto the bed and climbed on top of me. I told her I could see strangers peering in, but that just made her bolder and more passionate. You know what? As it turns out, I'm a big fan of having sex with the blinds up, too."

In silence Says Howard, thirty: "Actually, this may sound crazy, but one of my favorite places to have sex with my wife is at my in-laws.'

We sleep in her old bedroom, which is right next to her parents' room, so we have to be super quiet. If the bed even creaks once or if I grunt, my wife puts her hand over my mouth and whispers, 'Shh-hhh.' Sometimes I'll start laughing, and she'll cover my mouth with her hands, and then we wind up giggling hysterically. The struggle to stay quiet makes the sex super hot, and it's an extra turn-on because she feels like a rebellious teen all over again, sneaking a guy into her bed with the lights out after dark."

Mission possible—lingerie Says Pam, thirty-five: "My husband's office is right around the corner from Victoria's Secret, and every now and then I'll call him up before he goes to lunch and tell him to stop off and pick me out something special for later. By the time he gets home, he can't wait for me to open the box. It's always something super sexy, like a mesh thong or a lacy v-string. And I think it gets him extra turned-on to know that he picked it out. He can't wait to see me try it on, and trust me, it isn't on for very long."

Says Ian: Pam hit a home-run out of the park because 1) men love lingerie and can't get enough of the stuff (need I say more?), and 2) men are very task focused. By sending your guy on a solo lingerie mission, you're not only getting him turned on by browsing at all the different possibilities and imagining you wearing them, but you're also building sexual anticipation and postponing gratification.

Mission possible—sex toys Says Janice, thirty-three: "My husband and I were never into sex toys, until I got a gift certificate to www.GoodVibrations.com at my friend's bachelorette party. I didn't think much of it at the time, but when I showed the gift certificate to my husband, he got really curious and eager. He asked me what I wanted, but the whole thing sort of embarrassed me. So I told him to go online and pick something—anything. 'Anything?' he asked. 'Sure,' I said, 'I trust you. So yes, anything, whatever turns you on.' Later that week, when I asked him what he ordered, he said it was going to be a surprise. To be honest, I was more than a little nervous. I mean, I'm not a kinky person. What if it was whips and chains or some kind of crazy four-foot-long dildo? When the box finally came, I was more excited than a six-year-old on Christmas morning. I didn't know what was going to be in there. But it turned me on to think that I was going to be at his sexual disposal and that I was going to submit to whatever he had ordered in that box. Do you want to know what was in the box? Well, I'm not going to tell you. But I will tell you this: We've since gone through that gift certificate and many, many more. And now we take turns surprising each other. And remember how I said I wasn't a kinky person? Well, I guess that depends on your definition of kinky."

Says Ian: By giving each other the license to explore their personal fantasies, Janice and her husband have opened up new realms of mutual pleasure and possibility! Sometimes a little naughty surprise can be the beginning of a whole lot more giving and getting every day.

Selecting and watching porn together Says Nicole, thirty-one: "It always pissed me off that my boyfriends were into porn, and I had this idea from college that porn was basically for sexually immature frat boys. Then one evening my boyfriend and I were at the local video store, and we found ourselves in the porn section. He kind of gave me this 'What do you think?' look, and, on a whim, I said, 'Sure, let's go for it.' We picked up a couple of funny titles—one was called *Hannah Does Her Sisters*—and I have to say it was sort of fun just browsing all the titles with my boyfriend, since it made me feel less alienated from the whole thing. And it turned out watching it was actually sort of fun. The video was really cheesy, and it made us laugh. But it was also pretty hot, and my boyfriend definitely got turned on that I was turned on. And we wound up trying some of the positions they were doing on the screen, just for fun.

Says Ian: Nicole is dead on the money shot. In addition to turning a guy's interest in porn from an auto-erotic experience to a shared one, watching porn together is also a great way to get comfortable talking about sex with your partner. After watching Hannah do her sisters, talking about, well, pretty much anything doesn't seem like such a big deal. But ladies, it's important to make sure you address any concerns or reservations you may have from the outset, so the experience proves to be a positive and mutually gratifying adventure for both of you, rather than a potential source of contention. If you're worried, for instance, that he may ignore you in lieu of the women on screen or think you may prefer completing your sexual journey unaccompanied by visual aids, discuss these possibilities ahead of time. Remember to use this as an opportunity to get to know each other's fantasies so it brings you closer together long after the movie ends.

Planning your own porn film, but not necessarily shooting it Says Kim, thirty-four: "I've always been the type of woman who craves sexual stimulation and gets bored easily. I'm completely comfortable with sex toys, and I enjoy watching porn, both with my man and on my own. I have no problem taking charge of my own sexuality, but I've definitely wanted to get, shall we say, more theatrical with my boyfriend. I wanted to role play and explore some domination and submission themes, but I couldn't get my man to open up and go there. So one day, when we were watching a porn film together, I turned it off and said we could do better. That's when he got interested. He bought an old video camera off eBay because I didn't want anything digital that could somehow find its way onto the Internet, and we planned the whole scene. It was really hot, a kidnapper/hostage scenario: Basically he kidnaps me, ties me up, and turns me into his sex slave. Then, when he's sleeping, I break free, tie him up, and exact sexual revenge. Can I be honest? Just planning the movie was really hot. We even bought props and a costume for me; I wanted to play a prissy heiress. And I got really excited. I got off on the idea of tying him up and doing him, something we'd never done before. When it finally came time to make the movie, I got nervous about the actual filming. So we decided to rehearse it without a tape in the camera. We've since done two more films, one of which we actually put on tape. But, to me, the best part was planning and, especially, rehearsing and, of course, working out 'the dramatic kinks.' "

Says Ian: Like the "I had a sexy dream" tip, making your own porn film is an exciting way to explore your fantasies without feeling judged. After all, if you're making a film about a kidnapper/hostage scenario, then you're just exploring those themes without having to deal with whether you really have domination/submission inclinations. Your own sense of identity or how your partner perceives you aren't on the line. And like Kim said, so much of the fun is in the preparation. Some couples really do enjoy making sex tapes. But you shouldn't do it if it winds up making you feel self-conscious or pressured. A dress rehearsal (make that *un-dress* rehearsal) can be just as fun.

Webcam Says Lila, twenty-seven: "I caught my fiancé downloading porn twice, and it made me angry, especially since I thought we had a great sex life. We're very open and affectionate with each other, and it bothered me that he felt like he needed porn. Then I bought a new Mac, and I received this e-mail from Apple about how easy it was to set up a webcam. That's when I got an idea: I decided to make my own Internet porn for my fiancé. I set up the camera and the web page in our bedroom and called him at work and told him he had to check out this website. Anyway, he went onto the webpage, and I have to tell you, my heart was pounding. I came out of the bathroom in a towel like I had just come out the shower and sat at the edge of the bed and pretended to dry off. Then I put on a pair of panties and one of his pajama tops and got into bed. I never once looked into the camera, but pretended to go about my business as usual, which just happened to include a vibrator. I had never done anything like that before, and it was exhilarating. After I was done, my fiancé called and told me not to move; he was on his way home. Later, he confessed that watching me do that was the biggest turn-on he'd ever experienced, and he made me promise I'd do it again."

Says Ian: Kudos to Kim for making the most of technology and one-upping the Internet porn stars. Something else that Kim tapped into is the thrill of exhibitionism and voyeurism, which figure dominantly in more than 80 percent of sexual fantasies. In fact, they're half of the big four: exhibitionism, voyeurism, domination, and submission. With those four poles to navigate, the possibilities for creative sexual exploration are virtually limitless.

Cell phone photos Says Hank, thirty-six: "Julie's always using my cell phone to take photos—mostly of our friends and us. But one day I got to work, and she called me to see if I had checked out the new photo series yet. I was in the middle of a meeting, but decided to give it a quick gander. Man, I couldn't believe what I saw. I was floored: a whole striptease. I don't know what got into her, but it was amazing. She asked me to erase them, and I said, only if you promise to send me more. Several times. I totally love the photos she takes because the angles are all funny, and she's laughing all the way through, making silly faces. . . . The photos capture that combination of beauty, boldness, and shyness that makes me love and crave her all the more. Sometimes when I'm at work and feeling stressed out of my skull, all I need to do is look at those photos of my little stripper, and I feel like the luckiest guy in the world."

Says Ian: Another winning way to make technology work for you! Hank's Tigress excited him by building new levels of surprise and novelty into their sex lives and taking sex out of the bedroom and into the office, creating a broader landscape of desire.

Chat room fantasies Says Amy, twenty-four: "I saw that movie *Closer* with Julia Roberts, and there's that whole chat-room scene between Jude Law and Clive Owen where Jude Law's pretending to be a chick. I thought it was hilarious, and I told my boyfriend, Brian, that we should try it—we're big pranksters, needless to say. Anyway, we signed up on a couple of chat-rooms and started creating these Internet personas—there's Wild Blondie, Cowboy Marcos, King Cream, African Queen, and a bunch of others. It's sort of a goof, but we have a blast, and letting our digital alter egos go wild is a real turn-on. It's all typing, but there are chat rooms where you can actually put up a webcam and be seen while you have sex. We're not sure if we're ready to go that far, but we're talking about letting Cowboy

Marcos and Wild Blondie make their on-screen debut and do some 'digital swinging.'"

Says Ian: Hats off, once again, to Amy and her boyfriend for using technology to bring them closer together rather than pushing them apart. And the best part of what they're doing is not the sex simulation, but the fun and laughter they're having along the way, allowing them to explore their fantasies safely together.

Erotic chores Says Steve, thirty-seven: "Lisa's always on me to wait until after dinner to start the dishes. I'm always up and washing plates, in a half-assed way, just to get it over with as quickly as possible, usually while she's still eating. I tried to tell her that most women would be thrilled to have a guy who wants to do the dishes, but not Lisa. On top of it, it drove me crazy when she would inspect the dishes afterward. Then she told me she was going to give me a lesson in dish-washing etiquette. And I told her there was only one way in hell I'd listen: If she did it naked. Well, would you believe it? There I was doing the dishes, and she comes in wearing only a thong, bra, and high heels and says it's time for my lesson. And, well, let me say, I listened. I scrubbed. I waited. I took my sweet old time and got that job done right. In fact, I've asked for a few follow-up lessons, just to make sure."

Says Ian: Couples spend too much time quibbling about chores and not nearly enough time eroticizing the mundane and making things fun. I can't tell you how many women have complained about guys who seem to want to have sex at the strangest times, "Like when I'm ironing or vacuuming and looking my worst!" The truth is that sometimes when you think you look like your worst, you actually look your best to us. So, make the most of it. And you'll be surprised how extremely happy we are to lend a helping hand.

Trimming/shaving each other's privates Says Cheryl, twenty-eight: "One day I was in the bathroom shaving my legs, and my boyfriend, Carl, asked me if he could shave them for me. It was really gentle and tender, and then he looked at me and asked me if he could shave more. I said, 'Sure, if you let me shave yours.' That was the start of a really beautiful (and sexy) ritual for us. We don't actually shave each other because it's too itchy, and I prefer to get waxed, but we do trim each other down there with a little pair of scissors. It's a total turn on for both of us. Carl gets totally hot being so up close to me and carefully trimming everywhere. I sit on the edge of a chair, and he likes to go down on me and finger me too, while he's doing it. And then he stands up, and I do him. It makes me crazy when I'm trimming him, and he gets harder and harder right there in my hands. We usually hop in the shower right after and have really hot, steamy shower sex."

Says Ian: Sounds like a plan! Shaving or, in many cases, just trimming each other's genital hair is a sexy, intimate experience. It requires trust and patience. Washing, drying, soaping, shaving are all extremely personal, private, yet nurturing acts, which are perfect for a sexy encounter. So why not make getting clean a little dirty, too?

The model Says Cheryl, thirty: "My fiancé, Simon, is a 'painter,' and lately I've been posing nude for him. He's done a beautiful series of charcoal sketches, and it creates a very powerful erotic bond between us. I even let him hang one on the wall, and it's a turn-on to know that people know it's me up there. He said I was so good at posing that I should sign up to model nude in an art class he takes on Wednesday nights. When he said it, he got this mischievous look in his eye, and I asked him if that was something that would turn him on—all those eyes on my body. He said it was, so I figured why not. Personally I thought it was a turn-on, too. If you've never posed nude in front of a group of twenty strangers, I say go for it. It was one of the scariest things I've ever done, but also the most exciting. Simon didn't tell anybody he knew me, so it was like this sexy secret just between us."

Role-playing Says Sue, thirty: "I once pretended I needed something in the hardware store. I wore a very tiny, tight black dress with nothing underneath and went in and asked for a hand-held shower massager. Of course, all the guys in the shop offered to help me find it, asking lots of questions about what types of pulsating massage I was looking for. Then my boyfriend walked in and offered to help me find it. I pretended like I didn't know him. He just came over and said he could assist me. After paying, I walked out of the store before he did. He told the guys at the store he was going to go back to my place to install it, and they high-fived him, which he said made it even hotter. Then he came over, and we hooked it up, and I showed him exactly how I liked to use it, still pretending we had just met. We even acted sort of different with each other, like total strangers. And I felt slutty for going home with someone I'd just met, which really turned me on."

Says Ian: A nice twist on the classic "stranger-in-a-bar" scenario, where you pretend to be a single stranger and let your boyfriend pick you up, much to the chagrin of all the other guys trying to do the same. Every errand has an erotic twist, and a trip to Home Depot will never be the same.

Around the world in eighty beds Says Adena, thirty-two: "Dan and I haven't actually been around the world in eighty beds, but that's our goal before we have kids. I guess we feel like we have a lifetime ahead of us to sleep in our own bed, so why not do it in as many beds as possible—with each other—while we have the chance?"

Says Ian: Now there's a show I haven't seen on the Travel Channel yet. The truth is that the easiest way to shake up your sex life and add some sizzle is to have sex somewhere new (as opposed to *with* someone new). And who says it even has to be in a bed? There are beaches, parks, mountains, not to mention kitchen tables and other horizons to be conquered.

For his eyes only, not necessarily Says Sue, again: "I had one boyfriend who liked to watch me masturbate in public, like on a train or in the park. He would sit across from me, in a public place, a library, a coffee shop, basically anywhere. And I would pretend he wasn't there and surreptitiously rub myself to orgasm, knowing he—and possibly others—could see. Then right when I was about to come, I would look directly into his eyes and smile."

Says Ian: This is a biggie for guys: watching women masturbate. And to watch her do it in public to boot is tantamount to winning the lottery. One woman I know likes to use those tiny silent remote-controlled vibrators at movies and give her guy the remote. For her, the whole challenge is having an orgasm while appearing to nonchalantly watch the movie. For him, the challenge is following the story.

Fellatio at an afternoon movie Says Gina, twenty-eight: "My boyfriend and I love to go to movies that have been playing for a while during a work day, knowing the audience will be pretty sparse. I begin touching him, stroking him slowly. And I always make sure he brings a jacket or something to throw across his lap. Then I lean over and take him into my mouth. We both have to be really quiet and slow. I make him wait until a really loud scene comes on before I let him come."

Says Ian: Ah yes, exhibitionism, always a good one. Love in the afternoon is always more fun when you get to do it in secret with dozens of people around.

Planning a threesome, not necessarily having one Says Heidi: "I know my boyfriend, Jon, wants to have a threesome with me and another woman, but I'm not really into doing it. But it's fun to talk about. Sometimes when we're out at a bar or at the beach, we look around and set our sights on a particularly sexy woman that we pretend we're going to try and have a threesome with. Jon loves to hear me talk about why I'd be into her, maybe it's her breasts or the way she moves or something about the look in her eyes. Then we talk about what we'd do with/to her. I have to admit it really turns me on. And, who knows, maybe one day we'll really do it. Until then, it's fun to think about."

Says Ian: This is a great way to explore the idea of a threesome; making it a fun and exciting game, instead of a threat or source of conflict, teaches you that the best way to deal with divergent desires is to make them converge!

NOW THAT HIS HEART IS pumping and his mind is racing, it's time to transition into the bedroom, or wherever you're going to have sex, and talk about building and sustaining arousal. As you may have observed, many of the aforementioned foreplay scenarios involve physical stimulation. But it is essential to note that in every case I've discussed, the physical component is secondary to the mental component. And where you've begun your sexy adventure is not necessarily where you're going to finish it.

S[t]roking His "Heart-on"

11

SEX IS THE MAIN way guys express their emotions. Making love is our way of saying "I love you" and truly feeling it, as well as really meaning it. While women generally deem closeness a prerequisite for engaging in sex, for a man, having sex is the main way of achieving a true sense of closeness with a woman.

Brain scans of men and women during sexual response reveal greater activity in men in an area of the brain known as the insula, which registers emotion and also rates the significance of physical sensations. So from a neurological perspective, it appears that mean are more likely to correlate the process of sexual response with an emotional response.

Men don't need to be in love to have sex, nor do they necessarily feel love during sex, but when they are in a committed relationship with someone they love, sex is likely to be the most genuine conduit for expressing love.

If a guy becomes sexually disconnected from his partner, he's also likely to become emotionally disengaged as well. And this, in turn, could leave him more vulnerable to infidelity.

Men also turn to sex as a means to resolve an emotional conflict, much to their partners' stunned horror. I cannot count the number of times I've had a woman complain to me about a boyfriend or husband who initiates sex after a terrible argument. Such was the case with one woman who complained, "He screams and shouts all evening, and then we get in bed, and he starts touching my boobs and kissing my back. He's made me feel so unsexy and bad and ugly, and then he wants to do it. What's wrong with him?" It was no surprise that when I spoke with the husband, he told me he was hoping that by making love, they could make up and reconnect.

Similarly, men are often startled to find that after hot make-up sex, their partners are still angry and don't have the same sense of resolution. Over and over I've heard, "I don't get it. We made love, and she's still angry and holding a grudge. How can she have sex with me and still be mad at me?" For guys, they've literally put the issue to bed; for women, the issue is still festering under the covers, keeping them awake.

· · · · · · · · · ·

Dear Ian,

My husband and I have been married for a year, and we recently had a baby. Ever since then, my sex drive has gone down, and we just haven't gotten back into a sexual routine. I'm afraid he [may] go off and look elsewhere. Am I just paranoid?

—Sarah, thirty-four, stay-at-home mom

No, you're not paranoid; you're intuitive. As a culture, we have this fantasy that having a baby is the most intense form of bonding that a couple can experience. But, in truth, most marital dissatisfaction begins after the birth of their first child. And it's not just lack of sleep or new routines that leads to marital woes: It's the sense of emotional alienation many guys experience.

Think about it: Post-birth, oxytocin levels in women are higher than ever, which facilitates an intense sense of bonding between mother and infant. Most women say they experience a feeling of falling in love with their baby, and this infatuation period often lasts as long the mother breast feeds, but very often longer. Yet increased oxytocin levels have a side effect of inhibiting a woman's testosterone level. (That's right; women produce testosterone, too—not as much as men, but the hormone still plays a strong role in a woman's libido.) So even after a woman has physically recovered from the experience of childbirth, she may be less interested in sex.

Many new fathers have told me how guilty they sometimes feel after their first baby's arrival. On the one hand, they're happier than they've ever been and would sooner lose their lives than see any harm come to their child or partner. On the other hand, they often feel like third wheels in their own homes. This sense of emotional disconnection is seriously amplified by the lack of sexual connection, which is why it's really important to find ways to make your marriage a priority and remain intimate. It's not about the sex; it's about the emotional connection that comes with sex, especially for men. You need to remain emotionally and, thus, erotically connected to your partner for the sake of the baby and the well-being of your whole family.

Granted, you may be tired, uncomfortable, or just plain exhausted. I know it isn't easy. Your breasts are swollen and leaking, and you feel fat! I know. *I know!* But finding ways to maintain the sexual connection with your husband, whether it's through intercourse, or kissing, or just plain fooling around, can mean the difference between staying happily married or becoming a statistic.

. . . .

Whenever I talk to men who are sexually bored or feel they're trapped in a routine, they usually say that sex has become mechanical and predictable. And when I ask them to drill down and elaborate on what they mean by routine or predictable, it invariably comes down to, "We know how to get each other off, but there's no emotional connection."

The trick to maintaining the emotional-sexual connection is not just changing the sex script and introducing new positions or techniques, but becoming more emotionally engaged before and after each intimate encounter: It's finding ways to let the feelings of connectedness you experienced during lovemaking flow into the rest of your daily lives.

More than any technique or position, emotional presence is the currency of great sex. And, as we've been discussing in regard to foreplay and sparking desire, this sense of emotional engagement starts outside the bedroom. So while you're getting into his head and stimulating his mind, here are some simple techniques for touching his heart.

Embrace Until You're Connected

Whenever I'm working in my office with couples, not only do I pay careful attention to their body language—how they're sitting next to each other, whether or not they're holding hands or touching each other—but also at some point in my initial sessions, I invariably ask them to get up and hug if they're open to it. An embrace is very telling and can provide a real snapshot of the overall relationship. It's always interesting to see how long a couple maintains contact during an embrace and who breaks first. Most of us don't know how to hug or don't really hug in a way that fosters a sense of connection.

It sounds simple, but hugging—really hugging—is hard work, so embracing until you're connected is an assignment I often give couples. Make a point of really hugging each other *at least* three times a day: once before leaving for work, a second time when arriving home, and a third time before going to sleep. If you do nothing else, hug three times—but truly hug. Recent studies have shown that all it takes is a single twenty-second hug to significantly raise oxytocin levels and leave you both feeling calmer and more connected. For more on this technique and how it's used to stimulate great success in sex and marital therapy, I encourage you to read the groundbreaking work A *Passionate Marriage* by Dr. David Schnarch.

The Present of Presence

One of the biggest obstacles to embracing until you're connected is the baggage of life itself. So often we're angry, hurt, or stressed out about something the other person did. Or we're carrying around conflicts from work, the strain of a long commute, or the fallout from an argument with a colleague, a friend, or family member. Intimacy with our partner starts to feel like a chore or obligation, something we simply can't get ourselves to focus on without feeling anxious or distracted. Life will never stop happening around us, and we have to protect our bond—from the rest of the world, each other, and ourselves. This means setting apart some time when we make an effort to let go of everything else except our connections to each other.

I'm always saddened by the degree to which we let the outside world intrude on our intimate lives. So many of us have televisions in our bedrooms or else rituals—like reading or going to bed at different times—that may help us unwind, decompress, or wrap up our days, but not to reconnect. Even worse is when couples bring their arguments to bed. I'm not saying that there won't be nights when you go to bed angry, but you don't need to continue your arguments in bed. I'm a big believer that the place where you regularly have sex (which for most of us is the bedroom) is also a place that as much as possible should be argument-free and present-focused.

But that sense of presence begins with you, not your bedroom, and starts with that feeling you get when you embrace until you're connected. Not only does being present enable you to let go of the past, but it also allows you to focus on the experience of being together and the subtle to sublime sensations of sex.

Eyes-Open Lovemaking

Sex and marriage therapist Dr. David Schnarch writes about making love with open eyes as a way of fostering trust, presence, and intimacy. In fact, the main reason the missionary position is cross-culturally the most popular and prevalent around the world is because of the degree to which it enables us to maintain eye contact. It can be the most powerful sexual position, especially if the emphasis is on pressing (pelvis to clitoris). But it can also be the most routine and least satisfying if the couple isn't really present. Most of us are making love with our eyes closed, both literally and figuratively. Whenever I've talked to men about their most powerful orgasms, invariably those orgasms involve looking: At a partner's body and facial expressions, but more importantly, into her eyes, up to and sometimes through the moment of orgasm.

Kissing

This eyes-open approach to lovemaking begins with kissing, and while David Schnarch actually advises couples to kiss with their eyes open and endure the awkward, initially uncomfortable pupil-dilation that comes from such close eye contact, I think, like the embracing exercise, it's important essentially to use kissing to get connected and present. So many books or articles focus on the art of kissing, and so many times I've heard men complain about kissing techniques. The same goes for fellatio techniques. Not that you shouldn't have a knowledge of technique based on an understanding of sexual response and physiology, but whether you're kissing, hugging, orally or manually stimulating, or having sex, you have to let intimacy, presence, and emotional substance drive technique. The more you actually focus on technique and what you're doing or how you're doing it, the more you close yourself off to intuiting and responding to the experience you are ideally striving to create in tandem.

Five-to-One Statements

Eminent marriage therapist John Gottman has spent a lifetime working with thousands of couples, researching what makes some marriages succeed and others fail. Gottman concluded, "It is the balance between positive and negative emotional interactions in a marriage that determines its well-being—whether the good moments of mutual pleasure, passion, humor, support, kindness, and generosity outweigh the bad moments of complaining, criticism, anger, disgust, contempt, defensiveness, and coldness." Those couples that succeed in their marriages enjoy an overriding proportion of positive over negative sentiment. But how do you ensure that? "All couples, happy and unhappy, have conflict, but the ratio of positive to negative interactions during arguments is a critical factor," and Gottman proposed that this ratio should ideally be five to one. While it's impossible to go through life tallying positive versus negative interactions, I've found that it's possible to intuit whether positive sentiment overrides. But just to make sure, finish off any argument or discussion by embracing until connected, kissing in an emotionally present way, opening your eyes, and saying something positive to each other.

As we move forward into building and sustaining sexual arousal through orgasm(s), remember that foreplay is not just about getting inside his head and heart, but ultimately keeping the two of them and the two of you connected.

Arousal, Part 1: The Hands-Off
Secret to Hands-On Heat

NOW THAT YOU'VE CAPTURED his head and warmed his heart, it's time to lay hands.

Sex therapists often tell patients to think of arousal as a process that unfolds on a scale from one to ten, with the upper parameter representing orgasm. But in my professional experience, I've found that the idea of a one to ten "arousal arc" generally overestimates the male trajectory of sexual response: Male arousal more typically unfolds on an accelerated scale of, say, one to five, with one being low-level arousal, two and three resulting from direct genital stimulation, four being the moment of ejaculatory inevitability, and five being orgasm.

Or, to put it another way, as the founding editors of *Men's Health* magazine, Stefan Bechtel and Laurence Roy Stains, so succinctly put it in their book *Sex: A Man's Guide*, "Studies show that three-fourths of men are finished with sex within a few minutes of starting. But women often need fifteen minutes or more to become sufficiently aroused for orgasm. And therein lies a world of rage, grief, and airborne pots and pans."

Remember that guys tend to be orgasm-focused rather than pleasure-centered, so in extending his scale and taking him from one to ten, as opposed to just five, you have to first and foremost focus on the low-level arousal that often gets overlooked during sexual interaction. This means touching, nibbling, teasing, or, in other words, building excitement *without* primary genital stimulation. If you have any doubt whatsoever about the wisdom of this advice, just think back to how you felt when your annoying ex-boyfriend grabbed at your boobs or crotch, only to be stung with irritation when you instinctively pulled away. Now, if he had first offered a gentle shoulder rub or kissed the nape of your neck and whispered something naughty in your ear, things probably would have taken a far more satisfying turn.

I'm here to tell you that regardless of what you may think men want, we enjoy being touched, wanted, and seduced too (even if we're not accustomed to these forms of sensual stimulation in a sexual context). And I'm not talking about just flashing him a g-string or bit of cleavage (though it never hurts). I mean something that makes *him* feel desirable, wanted, relaxed, and physically charged. If you want to slow things down, you have to start by showing him that it's okay for him to kick back and enjoy the ride.

The experience of touch during sex is especially crucial to men because sex is one of the only situations in which guys actually give themselves permission to touch and be touched, and, even then, we remain plagued with a sense of guardedness. The truth is that men love nongenital-based touch, but we're inhibited, sometimes even feeling guilty, when it comes to asking for physical comfort in a sexual context. This ambivalence, as we discussed earlier, often stems from a number of underlying causes: a male sense of compunction to take the lead in sexual interactions, a discomfort with submitting to a woman or abdicating control, a sense of emasculation when not focusing on performance and penetration, and embarrassment at wanting to be stroked, flattered, and doted on (desires typically considered feminine).

Relaxation is the key to arousal, so in this early stage, when you're taking him from one to five, instead of focusing on turning him on, per se, focus on calming him down. Think about it: If stress inhibits erections, then it stands to reason that relaxation does the opposite. It promotes arousal.

When men are stressed out or anxious, blood flow is naturally redirected into the limbs as part of the primitive, hard-wired, flight-or-fight system. This is one of the reasons men often experience erectile difficulties when they're stressed-out or anxious.

Relaxation is the key to redirecting blood flow into the genitals. That's why men often get hard when they get a massage: They're not turned on, just simply relaxed. Most good masseurs know this, and rather than interpreting the spontaneous erection as a sign of sexual desire, they take the tumescence as a sign that they're doing their job well.

Another similarity between the sexes is that men also have different qualities of orgasm with varying degrees of intensity.

There's a wonderful passage in Norman Rush's novel *Mortals* in which the narrator recounts his wife's description of an orgasm, or rather, in her words, "what it feels like when you come really hard":

Well, part of what it feels like is this, that you're just a drop of oil on a white tablecloth, just a tiny, still drop of oil, and then in a flash you're expanding outward in every direction, evenly, turning into a stain, a little drop expanding into a bright stain that covers the universe.

Sounds pretty intense: And men, like women, have the propensity to achieve a more expansive, fully encompassing orgasm, what I call a "global" orgasm. Although, more often than not, they wind up experiencing a contained penis-based orgasm, a "local" orgasm, which may be sharp and pleasurable but lacks the fiber-tingling full-bodied resonance of its global brother. He may be coming but, to borrow the phrase, "is he coming really hard?"

Probably not: With an already compressed process of sexual response, coupled with a genital-focused approach to physical stimulation, men do not typically develop particularly high levels of myotonia (sexual muscular tension) throughout their bodies at the point of orgasm. The sexual tension is localized in the pelvic area and even then is inhibited by protections endemic to the region, which were discussed in Part I. Sure, it still feels good—that's the nature of orgasms. To quote Dr. Drew Pinsky, of *Loveline* fame, "Sex for us is like pizza, okay? You put anchovies on it, you put pineapple on it—all of it's good." True enough, but just as there's a difference between good and great pizza, there's a big difference between coming and *coming really hard*, and if you want him to experience the latter (a global orgasm), then you can't act locally. But when it comes to stimulating arousal, most women do exactly that: They think and act with one point in mind: the penis.

Women are just as culpable as men for perpetuating a narrow-minded penis-focused approach to sex, often gauging their own desirability by the speed and girth of a guy's tumescence and focusing primarily on his erection as a way of increasing this excitement. Sure, a hard-on can be a turn-on, but an erection is more than just a means to an end; it's part of a broader, holistic pleasure system. For a woman to focus solely on the erection as an indicator of arousal is as naïve as the guy who focuses narrowly on vaginal wetness as a sign of female sexual readiness. An erection may be a byproduct of arousal and certainly indicates a physical ability to perform, but that doesn't mean it has to be the focus of your arousing—at least not yet.

The first step in allowing him to relax and enjoy is alleviating his perceived pressure to be hard at all times. Showing your guy that you want him to enjoy the incredible (often new) sensations of sexual arousal without regard to his ability to pop and sustain a boner will ultimately allow him to relax and experience a shattering global orgasm.

So with a focus on building a strong foundation of arousal and keeping him in "the zone" (one to five), here are some tips for thinking and acting globally.

Get Him Naked

It's called "socks-off sex," and you'd be surprised how many guys are content to leave them on, along with other articles of clothing. Why are guys so resistant to getting naked? Most would say they don't have an issue: They're just lazy or else they get so caught up in the heat of the moment, they can't be bothered to get completely undressed; or some may simply say, "Why bother to do more than unzip my fly and pull my pants below my waist?"

But these are the very behaviors we need to change. Men *do* get lazy and stuck in those same old musty sex scripts. Men *do* get caught up in the heat of the moment—that's the accelerated process of arousal I've been talking about. And most men *do* focus primarily on direct genital stimulation and fail to respect the role other parts of the body (and mind) play in the arousal process.

Clothes-on sex is closed-off sex. It is the epitome of the localized orgasm. So when he gets completely naked, you're immediately subverting all of these bad behaviors. But, more than that, when a guy is totally naked, not only is he more physically receptive to pleasure (after all, the skin is the largest organ of the body, with a surface area of eighteen square feet), but he's also more liberated, vulnerable, and open to receiving pleasure. Men can have sex with their clothes on, but they can only make love with their clothes off.

Enjoy the Receiving End

Most of the time when we think about sensual touching, we think about giving rather than taking pleasure. This is especially true of women, who are socialized to put male pleasure ahead of their own. In my experience working with couples, I can unequivocally say that women are much more comfortable giving than getting and would often fake an orgasm rather than feel like they're inconveniencing their partners with their own "selfish" desires.

But women should realize that touching for their own pleasure, touching in an effort not to give but to take is not selfish at all: When you touch for your own pleasure, when you touch to turn yourself on, it will naturally turn him on. So don't focus on what he's feeling; focus on what you're feeling, and you'll both end up feeling good.

Tie Him Up

Render him lovingly helpless. Allowing him to revel in his willing-ness to submit to your lead is both liberating and erotically intoxi-cating, as male submission and bondage remains tinged with taboo. But exploring sexual domination is not about being kinky, but rather taking enjoyment in being the top to his bottom and feeling confi-dent that your enjoyment is a product of his.

When he's tied up, you're in control. It's a chance for him to re-main relatively passive while you direct the action. And that's both extremely exciting and relaxing (as discussed earlier), relieving him of an enormous sense of pressure to perform and dominate. Over and over, men tell me how being tied up figures into their fantasies.

It's not about how you do it or the extent to which he's actually tied up, but rather the symbolic nature of what you're doing. If you don't want to go out and buy handcuffs, try a bra or stockings. Thigh-highs are especially useful. His leather belt, an old tie— almost anything can do the trick. Just like getting him completely naked, restraining him helps him get to a place where he's vulnera-ble, exposed, open to new experiences, and receptive to a more ex-pansive sense of pleasure. It allows him to submit to the glorious sensations of being touched, wanted, and teased. Not being able to move forces him into his body, while not being compelled to per-form frees up his mind. You can't get more global than that: It's the full-body politic.

Be sure to explore his entire body and all of its untrammeled erog-enous zones extra slowly. It's all about teasing, taunting, and tantaliz-ing. Make him crazy with sexual frustration. But if you're new to the world of playful restraint, then take heed of some basic cautions:

- Don't bind him too tightly, as you don't want to damage any nerves or blood vessels. So tell him to pay attention to any signs of numbness.
- Never leave your partner alone while he's restrained.
- If you're role-playing while restraining—captor/captive, mistress/servant, teacher/schoolboy—establish an arbitrary "safe word" (such as "kumquats") to cease the action immediately.

Always end a session of restraint on a note of intimacy. After you untie him, make sure to hug, cuddle, snuggle, and kiss. Guys often feel very emotional and vulnerable after being tied up and want to feel loved and protected. Savor the moment for all its worth, both for the sexual power before and the tenderness after.

. . . .

Dear Ian,

My boyfriend and I recently started sharing fantasies, and it's been really liberating: We don't judge each other, nor do we feel a pressure to act them out. But many of my boyfriend's fantasies have included scenarios where I dominate him, like one where he told me that he fantasizes about me tying him up and spanking him. I asked him if this was a situation in which he'd like to turn fantasy into reality, and he smiled and nodded his head. Now I'm sort of freaking out. It's one thing to talk about a fantasy, but I've never tied up a man, or spanked one for that matter. What do I do?

—Rachel, twenty-nine, legal editor

First of all, congratulations on using fantasy to build excitement and newness and sustain a more satisfying sex life. So many fantasies go awry in their transition into action, so I think it's important that you don't feel pressured to do anything that makes you uncomfortable. The spirit of nonjudgmental sharing you've established with your boyfriend is far more important than gratifying any one particular fantasy.

That said, if you are curious to explore domination with your boyfriend, know that you're not alone in feeling a sense of hesitation. Women are very often socialized to be accommodating and sexually submissive to men, so it only makes sense that you may not be completely comfortable with playing the dominant role. Take the time to talk to your boyfriend in greater detail about the domination fantasy he'd like to enact and make sure you're both comfortable with it. Talk about the activities you're going to engage in. One of the problems with domination fantasies is that they're often so general— "Dominate me; I'll do anything you want." The more specific you get, the better. Decide on the activities you both find sexually exciting, and also talk about the activities that you're not necessarily excited by, but open to trying. Also talk about the activities that you're definitely not comfortable with and take them off the table.

For example, maybe he's fantasized about you spanking him, and you're comfortable doing this with your hand, but not with a paddle. You'll find that out by talking through your fantasies together in a light-hearted, nonjudgmental way; you'll be able to chart the terrain to greater sexual intimacy, regardless of what you wind up doing. You'll also develop greater trust, facilitating an endless array of new fantasies to follow.

Make sure you feel encouraged and supported and that the environment is trusting and stress-free. Don't set your expectations too high: My professional experience has shown me time and time again that fantasies, when acted out, rarely meet the sense of sexual excitement and gratification we expect. This is especially true of the first time we try something completely different. However, I've met scores of women who have really enjoyed, sometimes unexpectedly, the power of being on top and end up getting more out of the experience than just sexual thrills.

One woman I counseled was in a marriage where she was emotionally submissive and felt as if her husband held all the power. By exploring domination in the bedroom, she was able to redevelop a sense of confidence, assertiveness, and self-esteem that helped her to do the same outside the bedroom. On the flip side, her husband, the CIO of a Fortune-200 company, was finally able to relax and relinquish control, gratefully serving his wife's unwieldy sexual demands and taking his pleasures as she saw fit to bestow them. He, for one, was thrilled to rediscover this self-assured side of his wife, as it reminded him of the woman he'd fallen in love with many years ago, when they met at business school. They have been far happier for it, both individually and as a couple, and their sex life has never been better. Which goes to show that sometimes acting out a sexual fantasy or playing roles can help you take action and subvert real-life roles where you least expect it.

Blindfold Him

This introduces an element of surprise and gets him more attuned to what he's feeling. Chances are he will try to catch a glimpse, but that's all the better. Most men are visual creatures, so it will build tension and allow him to focus on the sensual and physical, while making him all the more desperate to get a good look at you after.

Also, men are so hard-wired to get aroused through visual stimulation that hobbling this sense allows his other senses—touch, taste, smell, and hearing—to *come* center-stage.

The Joy of Massage

Massage his feet, head, toes, neck, even fingers. We've talked about the role oxytocin plays in women as the cuddle hormone, but men have an equivalent hormone, vasopressin, which is also released during touch. This hormone tempers testosterone and helps him feel calm, relaxed, and connected, which is why it's informally dubbed the monogamy hormone. Dr. Theresa Crenshaw, author of *The Alchemy of Love and Lust*, wrote, "Testosterone wants to prowl; vasopressin wants to stay home." In the long run vasopressin plays a role in fostering his sense of paternalism, but in the short-term, the more you focus on touch, the more he's going to feel calm and connected to you. Massage also boosts circulation, which is essential for arousal.

Here are just some of the rave reviews I've heard from male patients whose partners have incorporated massage to foster greater sensual intimacy.

"I love a good firm, foot massage—it totally relaxes me: stretching my toes, kneading the skin in between them, it's a total turn-on when she sucks my toes, too."

"Nipples. Bite them, pinch them, tickle them, and nibble them—mine are more sensitive than my wife's."

"Fingernails on my back drive me crazy—I love a good back-scratch."

"I like to have my calves worked. My girlfriend holds my leg steady with one hand and really works it up to the knees."

"A good scalp massage is totally invigorating. I also love it when she puts a really hot washcloth on my face while she massages my scalp."

As you're massaging him, remember that his entire body is an erogenous zone, and many areas—like the earlobes, eyelids, and nipples—are rife with sensitive nerve endings.

Work His Pelvis

As we discussed earlier, men's genitals grow outward. From an early age, boys intuitively protect them. But over time, this instinctive desire to protect his privates manifests itself as a permanent sense of inwardness, a physical pulling in that ultimately extends to the entire pelvic area. According to Dr. R. Louis Schultz, "The muscles at the base of the penis may pull the organ in with habitual contraction.

Most women generally approach this area cautiously and briefly, as a pit stop before direct genital stimulation. But make this area a stop in its own right and open up his pelvis.

To get into the groove, take these basic principles of full-body massage and apply them creatively to his pelvis.

- **Effleurage:** These are long, stroking movements, which are performed using the flat of the hand or fingers by gently gliding your palms across his skin and then gradually putting your body weight behind the glide.
- **Petrissage:** These movements involve kneading, rolling, and the pulling of his skin. Begin with your fingers point-

ing away from you, and press down with your palm, while grasping his flesh between your fingers and thumb.

- **Tapotement:** These are fast and stimulating percussive movements that include cupping, hacking, and pounding (also called pummeling). While cupping, gently curve the hands to make a loose-cupped shape, bending at the knuckles while keeping the fingers straight and firm. While gently pounding (or pummeling), loosely clench your fists, keeping the wrists relaxed. Stroke your partner with either the outer edges of the loose fist or the front of the knuckles.
- **Friction.** Using your thumb, fingertips, and knuckles, apply direct pressure to a particular site of muscular tension. Lean gradually into the muscle and slowly deepen the pressure. Press for a few seconds, then release.

If you're interested in learning more about how professional Rolfers approach pelvic massage, I encourage you to read Dr. Schultz's eye-opening (wait till you see the photographs) guide for practitioners, *Out in the Open: The Complete Male Pelvis.*

Turn Him Over

Make sure to work his buttocks, which hold a great deal of tension. *Many* guys have a hands-off attitude about being touched in this area, but there's a big difference between massaging the buttocks to relieve tension and sensually massaging the anal area. Later we'll talk about direct anal stimulation to enhance and deepen the pleasure of orgasm, but for now, we'll focus on relieving tension.

Use a tennis ball to add some posterior pizzazz. By rolling a tennis ball along his back, you can give him a good massage, but the tennis ball is also a great way to get him comfortable with your exploration of posterior regions. Rolling a tennis ball along the lower half of his buttocks is a great way to take a hands-off hands-on approach to the more sensitive areas around the anus, like the space between his butt cheeks, as well as his perineum and anal entrance. You'll activate and stimulate the nerve fibers without transgressing boundaries that he may be uncomfortable with, at least for now.

Keep It Hot

Literally. Sex, especially vigorous, sweaty sex, stimulates the production of steroid hormones, tiny molecules like testosterone and estrogen that contribute to desire and arousal. Says psychologist Cameron Muir of Brock University in Ontario, Canada, on the virtues of sweating during sex and pursuant testosterone release: "The concentration is more than ten times higher, and that concentration is almost as high as the concentration doctors would prescribe for women to enhance the libido."

A S YOU FOCUS ON BUILDING arousal, don't let his erection or semi-erection distract you. Depending how well you manage to slow him down and relax him, you may notice his erection is semi-hard as opposed to being rigid-hard. He will probably need direct stimulation to get him fully rigid-erect.

Which brings us to the next stage. . . .

Rubbing Him the Right Way

S O, PASSIONISTAS, if you were to watch a guy masturbate in slow motion, what, precisely, would you see?

1. Well, you would probably see him engage in nonrhythmic manual stimulation, sometimes referred to as filling, because this form of light unfocused touch facilitates the filling of his penis with blood and its transition to tumescence from a flaccid or semi-aroused state. To get himself hard, he may:
   - Tap lightly along the shaft of his penis (as though he were playing piano on it with his index and middle finger).
   - Squeeze the glans (as though he were checking the ripeness of a melon), and gently stroke the frenulum and corona, where the glans meets the shaft.

- Grasp the shaft and shake it.
- Massage his testicles; pinch the scrotal skin; press, stroke, and graze his perineum and anal area.

The length of time it takes for this phase of filling to unfold ranges widely from man to man and is dependent on many factors: his level of arousal at the start, his age, the last time he ejaculated, and his overall sexual fitness. Some men like to linger in the filling phase and enjoy the feeling of becoming hard, while others will do the bare minimum to get to the next stage of arousal where the sensations are more intense.

2. Once he's even minimally erect, he will likely grasp and clasp his penis: If he's a rightie, he'll use his left hand to firmly grasp the base of the shaft and stretch the penile skin down toward his scrotum. This stretching taut of the penile skin significantly increases the sensitivity of the frenulum and glans as he forms a ring with his thumb and index finger and clasps just below the corona. Rhythmic stroking of the frenulum and glans increases blood flow to the penis and facilitates the build-up of sexual tension required for orgasm.

This sexual tension will manifest itself throughout his body, and many men will break from stroking the frenulum to squeeze their nipples or touch other parts of their body. While rubbing up and down along the frenulum and glans, he may also break his clasp at peak moments of arousal to squeeze the glans firmly, which will momentarily force blood back down out of the glans and consequently slow down the path toward ejaculatory inevitability while heightening sexual tension and building propulsive force.

3. As his levels of arousal build to a peak, he will experience the first of a series of pleasurable orgasmic contractions. Most men recognize this first contraction as the point of ejaculatory inevitability and take this as an intuitive signal to increase frictional massage of the frenulum and glans and tighten the grip on the base and shaft.

4. As the pleasurable orgasmic contractions propel semen through the urethra, he will retain his tight grip on the shaft and continue massaging the frenulum and glans, maximizing the pleasure and stroking through the orgasm and its first expulsion of ejaculate. He is likely to increase the force of stimulation to augment ejaculatory expulsion. Before finishing, he will squeeze or tap on the frenulum to expel the last pleasurable drops of semen before the tension in his body subsides and his penis returns to a flaccid state.

What I have just described is a four-part process of direct genital stimulation.

1. Filling
2. Grasping and clasping
3. Stroking and squeezing to ejaculatory inevitablity
4. Stroking and squeezing through orgasm and ejaculation

As his partner and Passionista, you need to be able to do all that and more. By all that, I mean you need to get attuned to his individual process of arousal and learn how to use appropriate levels of stimulation at each stage to maximize his pleasure and orgasm.

For example, though women often complain to me that their partners are too fast and furious when it comes to clitoral stimulation, according to their boyfriends and husbands, women also "jump the gun" and rush too quickly into heavy rhythmic stimulation of the penis.

Other common gripes are that women often stop stroking or sucking too soon, lessening the pressure and consistency of movements at the point of orgasm, rather than stroking through the orgasm to maximize ejaculatory propulsion. Alternately, they often continue stroking well past ejaculation and comfort.

I've often heard men say that their well-meaning partners will apply a new sexual technique they've read or heard about, but do so mechanically without any regard to their partner's particular arc of arousal, focusing on form over substance.

Playing Your Hand

When Wanda came in to see me, she was positively frantic. Not surprising given that her fiancé, Bob, had gently informed her that sex was becoming B-O-R-I-N-G and that he was having trouble maintaining an erection. As a result, she had loaded up on French maid's uniforms, fish-net stockings, and stocked her nightstand with every book she could locate on how to give the perfect blowjob and have sex like a porn star. She'd spent hours practicing how to deep throat on countless dozens of innocent zucchinis (purportedly the best phallic instrument for gauging teeth marks). By the time she came in, her head was spinning with all the different "signature" techniques and positions she'd memorized. Yet, despite her impressive efforts, her fiancé's interest and erection were falling steadily. My sense was that she was too focused on pleasing him rather than actually connecting with him. So I gave her the simple assignment of placing her hand over his while he pleasured himself to get more attuned to his particular arousal process through all four stages of stimulation. At first she balked. "You mean you want me to give him a hand job?"

Like many of us, Wanda had placed too high a premium on sexual flash and novelty and had therefore dismissed manual labor as something he could do himself. But in truth, she, like many others, needed to start from the beginning, learning how Bob liked to be touched, from the expert: himself. Almost like learning how to swim, she needed to learn the basic strokes before she dove into deeper waters.

The upshot? Well, let's just say the zucchinis are back in their vegetable bin, and Bob is no longer bored.

In short, masturbation serves as a critical baseline for understanding your partner's unique arousal arc through all four phases of genital stimulation. But you will recall that I said that I want you to be able to do all that "and more." By more, I mean that the physics of male sexuality seem to tilt toward a conservation of energy: Men only stimulate themselves long enough to develop the requisite levels of tension necessary for orgasm—no more, no less. Creatures of habit and efficiency, they tend to follow a fairly straight line from start to finish.

Using his masturbation approach as a baseline for understanding his pattern of genital stimulation, you're going to move him through the process, but you're also going to diverge. Rather than merely facilitating his arousal, you're going to slow him down, thus forcing him to develop significantly higher levels of sexual tension than he would normally experience during self-stimulation or standard intercourse-oriented sex. In this way, you will be able to expand and heighten the parameters of his pleasure at each and every level of stimulation by introducing variety and unpredictability.

Fillin' Good

A S WE PROCEED with techniques for direct genital stimulation, the most important thing to keep in mind is how to integrate arousal with desire. When all is said and done, these techniques are intended to be inspirational rather than followed in a rote manner. Not only can and should lovemaking be improvised, but also the techniques are not nearly as important as the overall connection and spirit with which they are executed. That's what's cherished and remembered. Permitting him to kick back, knowing it's okay not to be in control (hell, you prefer him that way!), can be one of the sexiest experiences to a man accustomed to remaining in control. Make sure you let him know that you know what you're doing, you like what you're doing, and you intend to be doing it a damned long while regardless of how much he wants or begs for it.

You will take your sweet time, up until you decide that he's ready and worthy to come. That's being a passionista.

Remember that sex is ideally a holistic integration of emotional desire and intimacy, intellectual spark and creativity, sensual pleasure and physical arousal. The best sex fuses and builds on all these dimensions. And the way to achieve this with a man is to make him realize you are turned on by him being turned on, that you do not want to rush through it or let him take control. Let him know that you want to make him wait, savor, and enjoy; that you want to know exactly what he wants and plan to use it against him without mercy; that you will tease, taunt, tickle, nibble, suck, and stroke him until he cannot take another instant. You will take your time playing with him, and then, if he is very, very good and asks extremely nicely, *perhaps* in due course you will . . . set . . . him . . . free.

- The first touch to the penis sends shivers throughout the body, especially after the rest of his body has been amply aroused. Did you know that men produce significantly higher levels of testosterone when they are being touched by someone else as opposed to themselves? He may know how to touch himself, but his touch can never replace the connection, freshness, and unpredictability of yours. But very often, women don't take the time to touch; they go straight for the rhythmic stimulation, thinking that's what he wants or that's what it takes to build and sustain an erection. And while he may indeed want that rhythmic stimulation straight out of the gate and it may provide a shortcut to a powerful erection, your goal is to provide him with a new and varied sex script. So take the time to really touch and experience his response. This first touch is a vital part of the excitement and sense of connection you're going to forge. Style is borne of substance, and the most important part of being a responsive lover is just that—being engaged and responsive.

- Start with gentle strokes, and be exploratory. Remember your goal in this phase—whether you're using your hands, mouth, or vulva—is to fill and maximize his erectile potential and set out at a slow pace. He may instinctively want to speed you along and encourage you to grab his penis. Or, he may grab it. (This could be the ideal time to experiment with a bit of bondage, by tying his hands together.) Still, hold your ground and remain in charge. At this stage, you should not be engaging in rhythmic stimulation, but rather unfocused genital touch. At key moments, you may create an expectation of rhythm, but rather than pursue the rhythm, slow or even cease genital stimulation altogether for a few moments to build, rather than race, toward the next level of physical arousal.

- Think of his body as a vast erogenous landscape, one that throbs luminously from the heat of your touch. As you're generating heat in his genitals, you want to keep the other areas warm. Don't divert *to* the penis, but rather integrate and build connections and pathways to the penis from other areas. Stimulating two body spots together ignites a wider swatch of nerve endings and provides twice the erotic anticipation, *especially* when one of those areas is his penis. Focus on keeping his upper and lower body connected.

Some hot pathways (think of them as the major erogenous interstates connecting north and south) include: lips/penis, neck/penis, nipples/penis, and earlobe/penis.

Hands

- Lying comfortably next to him, drape your fingers over his penis and focus on light sporadic touching throughout the genitals. Use your fingertips to caress and lightly tickle or ever-so-lightly scratch, rather than squeeze or grab.
- With one hand, softly cup his testicles and hold for a moment. While cupping his balls, use your fingers to delicately massage the lower part of the shaft where it meets the scrotum. While cupping his testicles, focus on some of the upper body-lower body pathways already mentioned: Kiss or nibble his lower lip, whisper something sexy in his ear, nibble his earlobe, stroke his hair with your free hand, or lick or kiss a nipple. After engaging in these "filling" activities, you'll be able to feel the rush of blood to his genitals and see the change in his erection. Think of this position (cupping his testicles) as a place to return to after stimulating his penis. It's a place to maintain contact, but also to take a break from some of the more intense stimulation.
- Return to his penis, and this time apply deeper fingertip pressure. Think of yourself as a potter gently kneading a piece of clay. Take the shaft between your fingers and squeeze it from different positions: the sides (where you'll probably notice his dorsal veins swelling); the top and

underside; the lower part toward the scrotum, and the upper part below the head which encompasses the frenulum.

- Press the flat surface of your fingernails against the shaft. All of these different forms of pressure and textures stimulate the receptors in different ways and create different exhilarating sensations.

- As you touch the frenulum (the underside of the penis encompassing the area just below the glans), you'll probably notice a tensing of the body, a bucking of the hips, or a kegel contraction (as we discussed in Part I). This area, the frenulum, is often referred to as the sweet spot, and many men consider it the most sensitive part of the penis. It's typically the area that gets the most rhythmic stimulation during masturbation. Tease this area lightly: Starting at the tip of the head, use a single finger to lightly pet the entire underside of the glans and frenulum—like you're petting a cat between the eyes with a single finger.

Mouth

- When you use your mouth in the filling phase, focus on kissing, licking, and nibbling, as opposed to sucking.

- Again, think about what you're doing with your hands and how to continue that upper-lower body connection. Or simply use your hands to cup his testicles or graze the sensitive skin just below his navel. And, above all else, talk! Make eye contact. Physical arousal is nothing without some desire to go with it.

- Intersperse your finger work from above with light kisses.

- Gently nibble on the shaft—don't bite, but press your teeth against his shaft, as you did earlier with the flat surface of your fingernails.
- Place one hand under the shaft and lift his penis a bit toward your head as you gently nibble on it. Avoid clenching, squeezing, or rhythmically massaging. Rather, use your fingers to help his penis come to attention, and nibble as though you were eating straight from a plate.
- Add some tongue. A single ice-cream lick up the shaft and across the frenulum will send shivers throughout his body. But don't lick consistently. Keep it random and unpredictable. Think of this phase as the ultimate tease.
- Holding the base of the shaft with one hand, come in from above, press your tongue against his urethra and the tip of his penis. Make a tongue-to-tip connection. Now *slowly* begin to take the spongy head into your mouth. Stop at the edge (the corona), think of it as the edge of a cliff. Don't suck. Simply hold the head in your mouth and let it bathe in the wet warmth of your tongue. As you do this, use your fingers to gently squeeze up and down the shaft.

Vulva

- Use his penis to stimulate your clitoris. Lying next to him side by side and facing him eye to eye, take his penis in your hand as you would a vibrator and use his glans to gently massage your labia and clitoral head. Focus on using the top part of his head to stimulate yourself, which shouldn't be hard if he's taller than you and you're eye to eye. Do unto yourself as you are doing unto him: In other words, hold off on rhythmically massaging your clitoris. Rather, focus on the connection between your respective heads and hold the moment. If you do take his penis inside you, as with the previous mouth-technique, only take the tip of the glans in—do not go beyond the corona, and don't let him thrust. If you need to, gently grasp the shaft just below the head to ensure that he doesn't penetrate deeply. In this position, with the head of his penis against your clitoral glans, focus on the upper body connection. Kiss him; connect your heads, lower *and* upper.

- In the same position as above (side by side, face to face), gently push his penis downward so that it is horizontal and perpendicular to your vulva. Now move your body closer to his and press your labia and vaginal entrance against the top part of his shaft. Ride his shaft. In this position, your labia will enfold the top part of his shaft, applying pressure from above. Your clitoral glans will be nestled against his pelvic bone. Hold the position. Stay still. Focus on eye contact. Kiss, nuzzle him, nestle into him, talk to him, tease him, do anything but thrust. Let yourself get turned on. Build your own sexual tension. Take from him as you give. In this position, cross your ankles and press your inner thighs against his shaft.

Please, Squeeze, at Ease

This first phase of genital stimulation is one that usually gets short shrift as the tendency is to proceed straight to rhythmic thrusting, which heightens arousal but also the inevitability of orgasm. Think about ways you can linger in each phase. Use the above techniques as a general menu, but be sure to do a full-tasting menu, taking your time to savor each dish.

- As you *please* him (and yourself), end each technique with a *squeeze* of the glans. Approach the glans from the top and position its tip in the center of your palm. Now wrap the rest of your hand around the fleshy head and give it a good firm squeeze. This squeezing action pushes blood down from the tip of the penis and decreases his ejaculatory inevitability. Get into the habit of pleasing and squeezing him.
- The main thing is to try to stay attuned to where he is in the process of arousal. Is he doing everything he can to thrust, or is he allowing you to linger and indulge in this phase? Is he, indeed, filling, or do you feel it necessary to proceed to rhythmic stimulation? Follow his rhythm, pace, and unique arc of arousal. If he's seriously excited (which is likely), follow your squeeze with an at-ease. Break from direct genital stimulation and do something else. Kiss him, whisper in his ear, massage him. Tease him. Taunt him. Tie him up. Take a trip to the south side of town, and touch, lick, or *gently* finger the anus (if he'll let you). And, always, let him pleasure you. Or let him watch you pleasure yourself and make him beg to get in the last lick.

Is He Ready to Move on to the Next Stage?

- Does he seem to have achieved a full erection?
- Can you see the veins in his penis?
- Is he flexing his PC muscle?

- Is he seeking out rhythmic stimulation?
- Is his body starting to tense with the development of sexual tension?
- Most important: Are you turned on? Are you ready for more?
- Test the temperature of his arousal. Take his penis in your hands and engage in about ten seconds of nonfocused filling activities. Tease him; titillate him. Then give his penis one or two quick strokes from bottom to top. Did his hips buck? Did his heart skip a beat? Did his penis visually flick with a deep pelvic contraction?

If so, it's time to move on.

Arousal, Part 2: Rhythmic Stimulation

HIS TIME HAS NEARLY COME. But don't let him regain the reigns of control. You need to be sensitive to his rhythm and move with it, but not be controlled by it. During this all-important penultimate phase, you are focusing on building and expanding tension throughout his body. You are thinking locally, acting globally, as they say. You must be attuned to his local state of arousal and aware of how close he is to the point of no return, but remember that the more you work him up and diffuse the pleasure throughout his body, the more shatteringly intense his orgasm will be.

- Continue to intersperse and punctuate nonrhythmic stimulation with forceful rhythmic strokes that encompass the
  full length of his penis (shaft and glans).

- As you increase the pace of your rhythmic strokes, decrease the period of nonrhythmic stimulation. As you transition to rhythmic stimulation, start with, say, a ten-to-one ratio: After approximately ten seconds of nonrhythmic stimulation, hit him with a couple of solid rhythmic strokes. Then gradually work toward a five-to-one ratio. Now dispense with the nonrhythmic stimulation all together and focus on slow rhythmic strokes. The key thing to think about at this stage is *slowly* transitioning from nonfocused teasing, squeezing, building, touching, licking, nibbling, and manual stroking to actual rhythmic stroking.
- Pay attention to his levels of arousal. You will want to lead him close to the point of ejaculatory inevitability, but do *not* take him to the point of no return. The longer you can keep him in this intense state of peak arousal, the more gratifying his orgasm will be.
- Use the "squeeze, please, at ease" method described earlier to transition between genital approaches and to keep his arousal at bay.
- And, always, make plenty of eye contact, talk to him, ask if he likes what you're doing. Tell him you're going to make him wait. Remind him that you're in control and you love it. Let him fully enjoy the sensations of kicking back, letting go, relaxing, and experiencing every touch, lick, stroke, command, kiss, smile, slap, and nibble.

Hands

- Focus first on a simple grasp and clasp. Get yourself in a comfortable position, and firmly grasp the shaft of his penis at the base. Don't be afraid to apply pressure, I promise he will tell you if you're gripping him too tightly. Many women worry that they're hurting men when they squeeze tightly, while a common complaint from men is that women do not squeeze tightly enough when they are highly aroused. (In a culture where women fret over vaginal looseness and are chided continuously to practice kegels or even to consider extreme newfangled vaginal rejuvenation surgeries to tighten up, the reality is that a well-positioned manual clasp will serve the purpose more effectively.)
- With your free hand, use your thumb and index finger to form a clasp just under the coronal ridge, around his frenulum.
- Starting at the coronal ridge, stroke down to the base and then back up. Keep the movement slow and easy at first.
- Vary this long stroke with short strokes that are confined to the frenulum. Many men masturbate themselves to orgasm with these shorter, more rapid strokes.
- It may be time to add lubrication, particularly if you are emphasizing manual stimulation. While your own natural vaginal lubrication is the preferred choice, if it's not in ample supply, a water-based lubricant is your best choice. Oil-based lubes are not compatible with latex and whatever safe-sex precautions you have in place can also lead to

yeast infections. Silicone-based lubes last longer than water-based, but they're also harder to wash off and are incompatible with silicone (and therefore lots of sex toys).

- The simplest way to add lubrication into your routine is to squeeze some onto your hands and rub them together and get to work. When it comes to adding lubrication, less is more. But, remember, if you're using a water-based lube, keep the tube on hand, as it dries out more quickly. Too much lube may make matters too slippery and lead to more rapid stimulation. Some other fun ways to lube him up include dripping some on your stomach and letting him rub against you or dripping some in the cleavage between your breasts and letting him rub as you squeeze your breasts against his shaft. But take note: Stomach and cleavage rubs are also some extremely popular ways for men to thrust to orgasm.

- Once you've lubed him up, focus on slow, intense pressured strokes from the bottom to the top that go up and over the head.

- You can also loosen your clasp and go up and down over the head more briskly, all the while maintaining a loose clasp that barely grazes him.

- Rule of thumb: When using a loose clasp, increase the speed of your strokes. On a tight clasp, slow down. Genital arousal is all about the relationship between friction and pressure. When men masturbate, they tend to find a comfortable balance between the two in their strokes, but often will emphasize one element over the other to vary the quality of orgasm. An orgasm that comes from longer, pressured strokes may feel deeper, whereas an orgasm that comes from lighter, shorter strokes may feel more ticklish and propulsive. Both are intense. But one of the reasons that men often thrust violently during oral sex or intercourse is to compensate for insufficient friction or pressure.

- Lube up both your hands, sandwich his penis (head and shaft) between them and rub them together as though you were warming your hands. (The same can be done with your breasts. Douse some lube in your cleavage and push your breasts together, rubbing them up and down along the shaft and head of his penis, following the nonrhythmic to rhythmic stroke ratios we talked about earlier.)

- With a slightly dryer hand, get a good grip and wring his penis with both hands using the motion (but not the strength) you would use to wring out a towel.

- Remember to hold your grasp at the base of his penis— your grasp is going to help retain blood in the penis and heighten the quality and intensity of his orgasm. Additionally, use your free fingers to gently massage his testicles, pressing against his perineum or grazing his anal area. Feel free to break the grasp to engage his upper body, but remember to come back. (Chances are he won't let you forget.)

- As you "please," don't forget to "squeeze" and add an "at ease" at regular intervals. This is especially important during the rhythmic stimulation phase, as you could easily continue your stimulation straight through to orgasm. The squeeze and at ease will help you bring him close to the point of no return, without sending him over the edge.

Take a short break from direct genital stimulation altogether before transitioning into a different approach. Incorporate more teasing, tying up, and dirty talk here. Make him serve you by using his penis or tongue as your personal sex toy. Show him that you mean to make him wait, maybe even beg, and that you're in control—that you will not release him until you've had your fill of pleasure. Alternate between stimulating him and yourself. Continue to maintain contact, keep him close, but do not send him over the edge of ejaculatory inevitability.

Mouth

- In the rhythmic stimulation stage, your mouth is going to be most powerfully used in combination with your hands, with oral attention largely lavished upon the head and frenulum, the most sensitive parts of the penis.
- Maintaining a firm grip on his shaft, place your lips over the head and form a seal. By bobbing your head up and down over the frenulum, you will naturally create suction, and you can experiment with how it feels. Some men love suction, others find it uncomfortable, and still others are indifferent.
- Press your tongue against his frenulum and use the hand around his shaft to move his penis up and down and back and forth across your tongue. Dote on the frenulum. Lick it slowly, delicately, while maintaining a very tight grip on his shaft. Think of your hand as a blood-pressure sleeve that's increasing in pressure.

While maintaining your two-fingered grasp around the base, create a seal with your mouth and take in as much of his penis as you're comfortable with. Take heed: You *don't* need to deep throat. You can certainly do it if it's something you enjoy or think he may enjoy, but any stimulation you can provide from deep throating is something you can accomplish just as easily with hands and mouth. In surveys of men, deep throating is not a technique that features high on any man's wish list, except as a quick bit of novelty or fantasy. The last thing he wants is for you to be anxious or uncomfortable while stimulating him. It's more important that you stay engaged and attuned to the process. Most women enjoy performing oral sex on men, provided they don't feel anxious or like they're going to gag. They love the intimacy, the connection, and the power they exert, and the more strongly they feel about the man, the more intimate they consider the act. When women experience trepidation about fellatio, their anxiety usually stems from the following areas: Concerns about hygiene, fears of gagging, and discomfort (whether physical or psychological) about swallowing. So keep him clean, don't take more of him in your mouth than you're comfortable with, and if you don't want to swallow, then don't. Chances are he won't mind. Related to gagging, some women also worry about the violence of a man's thrusting, particularly as he gets increasingly aroused. When he's thrusting, it's called irrumation, as opposed to fellatio. During the latter, you're moving your mouth up and down his penis. You're in charge: You control the rhythm, pace, and pressure. In the case of irrumation, he's thrusting in and out of your mouth.

In any session of oral stimulation, there's likely to be a bit of both, but make sure, in general, you're in charge, and remember that men tend to buck and thrust when there's some sort of stimulation (either friction or pressure) they require to maintain arousal. As for swallowing his ejaculate, the main thing men enjoy is stimulation through orgasm. Many women stop at the point of orgasm, rather than stroking through the orgasm. Swallowing naturally provides that persistent stimulation, which is why men enjoy it. But if you don't enjoy swallowing (and *many* women don't), there are plenty of other ways to stimulate through orgasm and maximize his pleasure, with your fingers, breasts, and tongue. What's most important is to understand that men love being orally pleasured in a countless number of ways. There are many, many paths to sexual gratification, and no one approach is necessarily better than the rest. In fact, you should get out of the habit of taking the same path each time. What's important is that you understand the principles of pleasure and continually find new and creative ways to attune yourself to his pleasure with confidence. Your excitement and sense of control will be the most erotic aspects of any sexual interaction.

Intercourse

- As you did in the previous phase, use his penis like a vibrator or dildo. Lying side by side, face to face, eye to eye, take his penis in your hands and massage your labia and clitoral glans. Enjoy yourself; let yourself get aroused. Focus on taking pleasure, rather than giving. Use his body for your own enjoyment. Match your level of arousal to his. In controlling the sex script, you also need to take responsibility for your own pleasure. Being able to give pleasure is a relatively simple matter, but being able to take it is often a far greater challenge for many women.

- Do the slide, also known as femoral intercourse. Lube up his shaft, get on top, and let your labia enfold the underside of his penis. Slowly slide up and down his shaft. Lean forward slightly and press your clitoris against him.

- Lying side by side, push down his penis so it's perpendicular to your vulva and let your labia enfold him from the top. One way to vary the femoral intercourse described above is to squeeze your legs together and press your clitoral glans into his pelvis. Again, use your fingers to keep his penis in place. Let him thrust between your legs, while you grab and caress his buttocks.

- Get on top, and let him barely penetrate you—just the tip of the head. Now slide down to encompass his entire head to the edge of the coronal ridge. Hold the position. Now push down over the ridge to the heart of the frenulum and then back over the ridge to the fleshy part of the head. Work this area with small, slow movements, focusing primarily on the feeling of going up and down the coronal ridge.

- Either from the top or the side, penetrate deeply with a single thrust and hold the position for at least ten seconds. Massage your clitoris against his pelvic bone. Now very slowly pull up and out. As with the fellatio techniques we discussed, remember that you're in charge, you're leading, and you're the one doing the penetrating and thrusting. So try to focus on positions (like you on top or side by side) in which you can maintain a high degree of control.

- As you pull out from a deep thrust, squeeze your PC muscles (in other words, do a kegel) and tighten your vagina around his penis.

- Let him get on top and do the same thing. As he penetrates you, tell him to stay still and squeeze your PC muscles around his penis in rhythmic contractions, rather than letting him thrust. Control his movements by placing your hands on his butt. Hold the moment. Press your clitoris against his pelvis. Massage his buttocks and spread his cheeks a bit. Press his perineum and stimulate his prostate from the exterior. Tell him or prod him to slowly pull out and squeeze your PC muscles as he withdraws.

- When employing deep penetration, the point is to focus on single thrusts that are controlled and provide clitoral stimulation. The danger with any of these intercourse positions is that the session could easily spiral out of control and result in the sort of wild thrusting that produces lots of vaginal friction and his orgasm, but not yours.

- While somebody somewhere is attempting to work their way through the kama sutra, there are really only four major positions and then nearly infinite derivations. The four major positions are female superior (woman on top), male superior (man on top), side entry (face to face), and rear entry. Each of these positions offers their own unique attributes. The female superior position is the most consistent position for vouchsafing the female orgasm. When you're on top, you're not only getting direct clitoral stimulation, but you're also in control of the rhythm and intensity. You can focus on deep pressing more than thrusting, while also enjoying the feeling of being filled vaginally. Additionally, many men say this is their favorite position, not only because they know it's the one you're most likely to enjoy, but also because he can stimulate your breasts or simply lay back, relax, and enjoy the show.

Women are all too familiar with the feeling of a man climaxing and then collapsing on top of them, and the female superior position often offers a nice reversal of this dynamic. Remember that when you're in the female superior position, you can also use your hands for additional clitoral stimulation, or you can have him use his hands.

Additionally, many men have told me that they love using a vibrator to stimulate the clitoris when a woman's on top, or you can surprise him by whipping out your vibrator and using it on yourself. Men need to learn that rarely does unassisted intercourse (i.e., complemented by a hand, mouth, or vibrator) lead to female orgasm. The major downside of being on top is that many women are uncomfortable with their bodies and self-conscious about being seen. My advice is to turn down the lights, and get on top.

- In the male superior position, he's going to have more ability to thrust and achieve the momentum necessary for a really propulsive orgasm, so this could be a great position if you've already had yours and want him to have his. Many women enjoy getting their orgasm from the female superior position, knowing that his isn't far behind and then transitioning into the missionary position. But by placing your hands on his butt cheeks, you can hold him inside you and receive clitoral stimulation, while also massaging his buttocks. Like the female superior position and the side-by-side position, the missionary position is a great lovemaking position in that it affords body-to-body, face-to-face, eye-to-eye contact. It fosters emotional presence and offers a form of intimacy that is part and parcel of genuine ecstasy.

- Like the missionary position, side-by-side is a great one for making love. Because it's harder to thrust when you're each on your side, it also predisposes the coupling toward slower, deeper lovemaking. This can be assured when you wrap a leg over his and hold the position.

- Rear entry is a powerful position for many men. It lends itself to strong feelings of power and dominance and affords maximum thrusting for the propulsive orgasm. Many men find that they can only get past the point of ejaculatory inevitability from this posterior position. When he's coming in from behind, you're also likely to experience a comfortable pressure and stimulation against your G-spot.

- While there's no shortage of sexual positions for you to experiment with, don't let form overshadow substance or performance outweigh the pursuit of pleasure. Use these four basic positions—female superior, male superior, side-by-side, and rear entry—to explore, like points on the compass, the parameters of pleasure and intimacy. And by all means, switch positions throughout, ending often with oral or manual stimulation to orgasm, his and yours. There is no prescribed rule that says his penis must end up in your vagina when the sheets grow cold. Keep it hot and varied.

- Your vibrator isn't just for you. Boys enjoy toys as well, especially when you're using them on him. During oral or manual stimulation, put your vibrator on a low speed and press it against his shaft, frenulum, and head. You'll probably need to use both hands to encompass both the vibrator and his penis, unless you're using a very thin vibrator (such as the Rocket).
- Lower the vibrator against his shaft and simultaneously lick his frenulum, or use your mouth to create a seal around his head.
- Or use the vibrator when he's deeply penetrating you in the male superior or side-by-side position to stimulate his buttocks, anal entrance, and perineum.

Is he close to the point of ejaculatory inevitability (also known as the point of no return)?

- Does his body seem to be reaching a point of maximum tension?
- Are his testicles retracting toward his body?
- Has he entered the emission stage of ejaculation, as muscles close to the prostate begin to visually shudder?

- Has the spongy flesh of his head become even more tumescent as it fills with semen?
- Has he secreted that first drop of pre-ejaculate?

If so, he's about to go over the edge, and you need to determine whether you're going hit the brakes or step on the gas.

My advice?

Pump the Pedal!

O NCE HIS GUN has loaded (so to speak), help him focus on firing it for all it's worth.

- Once you've felt that spasm from the emission phase, which means he has crossed that point of no return, grab hold of his shaft and speed up and massage the base of his penis. The pressure on his shaft will intensify the pleasure of ejaculating, but the friction will increase its propulsiveness for an orgasm that is qualitatively more intense than an orgasm that comes from most forms of vaginal penetration alone.
- Alternatively, when he's at that exhilarating point of no return, why not use your mouth and hands instead? There's more than one way to skin a cat. The surprise, the change,

and the increased intensity of the oral and digital stimulation, which is easier for you to control than through intercourse, can provide a shock of excitement in addition to increasing the level of friction and pressure.

- Not that he doesn't love orgasms through intercourse—the only problem is that when you're in a position that's focused on deep penetration, pressing and clitoral stimulation, much of the sexual tension is being generated from the action on the base of the shaft. These orgasms can be deep, but may lack a top. In women's terms, it's like the difference between coming as a result of very fast, purely topical clitoral stimulation and coming as a result of slower clitoral stimulation plus deep penetration. You can and should squeeze your PC muscles while he's coming, and if you're coming too, he'll feel those vaginal contractions as well, but again this will add to the pressure, rather than provide friction.

- To compensate for any loss of friction and pressure, use your hand if he's on top or side-by-side to massage his buttocks, press his perineum, or play with his anal area. Remember the anus participates in the pleasurable contractions of orgasm and is filled with nerve endings. By pressing against his perineum, you're stimulating his prostate. Some men, at least at first, may find this pressure uncomfortable, while others will immediately embrace it. For many men, simply grazing the anal area (perineum and anus) with your fingertips is enough to add a quivering intensity of sensations to climax.

- If he's in a missionary or rear-entry position, he'll likely focus on fast thrusting to experience the friction against the frenulum and shaft. But, here, there's often a lack of pressure against the shaft. So, as he's coming, squeeze strongly on your PC muscles at the moment he makes his crucial thrust. Or, if that's too hard to control, try to bring your legs as close together as possible so that they are pushing against the sides of his penis.

Or give him an orgasm through a combination of your mouth and hands, providing an ideal combination of friction and pressure.

- As we discussed earlier, hold that pressure on his shaft—he may clasp his hand over yours to loosen or tighten the grip, or simply secure it. So take heed to his desires, and don't be put off or think you're doing a bad job if you suddenly feel a hand over yours.
- With your free hand, or mouth, continue to massage the frenulum. Many men say that there's nothing more exquisite than a tongue lapping against the frenulum at the moment of orgasm.
- His first spurt will contain the lion's share of ejaculate and will, by and large, be the most pleasurable. If you're giving him a hand job, you'll probably capture much of the semen on your hand, and if you're using your mouth, it's your decision whether you want to swallow, capture in your mouth and spit out, or let him ejaculate elsewhere.
- The main thing is to stroke through the orgasm and maintain contact.
- After his first spurt, loosen your grip on his shaft and also slow down your stroking of the frenulum.
- Now do the reverse of what we've discussed. Lighten your grip at the shaft, but intensify your clasp at the head. Focus

on one or two deep strokes of the head that will lead to the expulsion of more ejaculate. You may want to take your stroke halfway down the shaft and give it an intense stroke back up and over the head. Do this one or two more times to extract those final shudders and pause for a few seconds.

- Now take his frenulum between your fingers and give it a light squeeze to exact the last drop and exquisite shudder.
- Pause for at least half a minute, as the penis is extremely sensitive post-orgasm.

Use this period to connect with him face to face, eye to eye. Touch his face, stroke his hair, kiss him, hold him, connect with him. Those thirty seconds are his true afterglow, where he's seeking that loving connection.

The Butt Stops Here

THE BUTT OF MANY JOKES, the crack of many smiles, the der-
riere has been *rear*ing up in unexpected places: one of them
may be your bedroom. Whether this is cause for pleasure, laughter,
or downright alarm, from yours to his, it's important to broach the
issue with delicacy, understanding, and also some humor. So bot-
toms up!

As we discussed earlier, the entire buttocks is rife with nerve
endings, comprising the largest nongenital erogenous zone in the
male body. Even a superficial massage will extend his sensory experience beyond the familiar nerve endings in his penis for a deeper,
more embodied global orgasm, one he could never achieve on his
own. This can be achieved with the simple addition of pulsating
your fingers against his butt cheeks while taking him into your
mouth, with a few squeezes, taps, or slaps thrown in for good

measure. It can also be implemented to fire up the plain ol' missionary position by firmly gripping his butt in your hands to control and restrict his movements (thus, layering in a dominating nuance). Press your palms into his cheeks and apply varying degrees of pressure, using your PC squeezing and releasing techniques in lieu of thrusting, to remain in control. This will allow him to relax.

How much he will allow you to delve beneath and between the gated portals will depend, in large part, on your own level of comfort and sense of mastery (or should it be mistressy?). So, as always, make sure he sees that you know what you're doing and far more critically, that you like what you're doing, and that you want him to relinquish his will to your capable care. The more you are able to project a positive sense of excitement, pleasure, and adventure, the greater the likelihood he will open himself up to a richer, maybe even uncharted, experience. But before heading down yonder, do your best to abate any concerns you may have regarding hygiene. Better yet, make cleanliness an exciting part of your routine.

Strip him down to the buff, while you remain semi-clothed in lingerie and give him a shower or bath. Then slowly lather him up and wash him down from head to toe and everywhere in between. The warm water will help relax him (which is vital for a backroad excursion) and will focus him on his sensual enjoyment. You may also want to watch him wash himself, directing his strokes and telling him when he is permitted to start and stop. This will push his (and your) hot buttons by incorporating key themes of voyeurism, exhibitionism, and domination into the rinse cycle. Try tying his hands behind his back or blindfolding him while you wash him to layer in submission and round off the big four hot list.

Now that he's buffed and buff, it's time for a little dancing cheek to cheek. Most men will allow at least a bit of stimulation of their sweet spot, or perineum, which is the soft cushiony area located between his testicles and anus and is positively bursting with pleasurable nerve endings. By integrating gentle, tickling strokes of your fingertips when you orally pleasure him, you will increase his excitement tenfold. In fact, be sure to keep an eye on how close he is to the point of no return, so you don't move him too quickly through his arousal arc. You can also stimulate his sweet spot with a flickering tongue while you pleasure him with your hand. Again, make sure to remain decidedly in control. You may also want to incorporate the use of a small vibrator, by rubbing it up against his perineum (and watching him jolt with appreciation). Tell him how much you love watching him and making him wait. Give him confidence in your desire and ability to hold the reigns of control.

Continuing your journey, you may soon encounter a bit of resistance. Always respect his boundaries (especially, I may add, if you have your naughty boy cuffed, bound, or blindfolded), but remember that your own sense of desire, comfort, and control will best allow you to pioneer your way. If he will allow it, whether during a first encounter or subsequent journey, lightly stimulate his anus with your tongue or fingers. This area is extremely tender to the touch, so be careful or you will soon find yourself evicted and forcibly removed. Lick the outer ridge or rim of his anus—hence, the term rimming—or massage him gently with the cushions of your fingers (no pointy nails, folks!). That will make an ordinary hand job or blowjob a world-class adventure.

The final frontier of your journey is penetration, once again, if he'll allow it, and only if you, too, are comfortable and desire it. Second only to cleanliness, many women are resistant to the thought of penetrating their partners due to an odd societal stigma that equates anal stimulation with homosexuality and, hence, emasculation.

Homophobia notwithstanding, this association speaks volumes for our restrictive view of heterosexuality as predicated upon penile-vaginal intercourse. No part of the body belongs to any sexual orientation. Breasts are not the provenance of straight men, no matter how much they tend to think it, and asses are not the fodder of solely gay delights. I would ask you to look within yourself, rethink any pejorative conceptions you may have, and make a full-faith effort to reconceive your limited, limiting views of his body and your own to make it a fully navigable, wholly sensual, and exquisitely sexual domain for endless exploration and pleasure.

That said, if you and your partner are ready to continue your trip, you should combine finger and mouth stimulation in initiating anal penetration, as it provides necessary lubrication as well as intensely pleasurable sensations. Get attuned to his rhythm and place a single cushioned finger (again, no nails, ladies!) on his anal opening. Only when you feel him relax and open (trust me, you will), gently nudge your finger in and let it rest there, motionless. Continue to lick his perineum and anal ridge while slightly vibrating your finger, without moving it in further. When you feel him open more (which he ideally will at some point), gently nudge it in further. Continue slowly until you have inserted your finger a full two inches into his anus, pressing forward against the wall of his perineum: Congratulations friends, you have hit his G-spot. Once he is comfortable, you can continue to penetrate him while you suck and stroke his testicles, perineum, and penis until he is ready to luxuriate in a breathtaking orgasm. As always take your time and make him wait. I heartily suggest you keep your finger in his anus at first, rather than pushing it in and out. Move it slowly back and forth and side to side, tapping on his G-spot. You may add longer penetrating strokes in and out for variety when he is clearly ready or incorporate a small vibrator or butt plug. But remember, his G-spot is inside, so don't go Rambo on him and do unto him what he may have done onto you. We're not going for the thrust here. To make this not only a spectacular, but also an emotionally meaningful surrender to your power, be gentle, sensitive, and utterly unyielding of control. Remember, having him ask or beg, tying him up, pinching his nipples, and stroking his chest will help make this an epic climax that he will never forget and will want to repeat, with new and exciting twists (literally and figuratively).

Also, and this is key, *he may lose his erection.* Some men, for a combination of psychological and physiological reasons, cannot maintain a full erection when penetrated. *Do not* let that inhibit your journey or make him self-conscious about it. Keep on trucking, sistas! Make him wait. Build the tension throughout his body. And when he does finally explode into orbit, he will most definitely thank you for it many times over, buried head first between your thighs—that is, once he recovers from his post-orgasmic stupor.

Conclusion

OKAY, SO YOU REMEMBER that guy Charlie I was telling you about in the Introduction—the one with the killer sex life who's been married with kids for nearly ten years?

Well, I finally sat him down in my office one day and asked him to tell me his secret: What exactly did he and his wife do to keep the fires burning so intensely? And you know what he said?

"We don't *do* anything, doc."

"What do you mean you don't do anything?"

"I mean, sure we *do* stuff, but it's not about what we do."

"Then what is it about?" I asked.

"Let's see, how can I describe it?" Charlie began. "Well, it's like a few nights ago, I was watching this show about how the universe is expanding. Did you know that was Einstein's biggest failing? He thought the universe was static. So, when he finally did figure it out, he said it was the greatest blunder of his life. . . . Well, I think that's the biggest blunder we make in our relationships—we assume things are static and don't let ourselves expand with the universe. I dunno. I'm not sure if I'm making any sense here."

"Actually, I think you're making a whole lot of sense, Charlie. Sex is about expanding who we are, what we want, and what we think we want in the most incredibly intimate way."

Charlie nodded.

Suddenly, I thought about the woman on the shaky bridge. The psychologists who'd conducted that study went on to hypothesize that falling in love was a process of self-expansion, that first powerful bang when you're staying up all hours of the night talking and touching, getting to know each other's likes and dislikes, disappointments and aspirations. And it's not simply that you're falling in love with the other person; it's that it allows you to fall in love with yourself through their eyes as well, to rediscover yourself, to question who you are and, what you want. And it all happens at such a frenetic speed, it's like an electric current recharging your brain.

But once couples get to know each other, they usually stop asking as many questions of themselves and each other, and that thrill of rapid expansion decreases, resulting in a precipitous drop-off in levels of satisfaction and love. If, however, they continue to engage in mutually expanding activities, they can continue to experience that sense of awe and discovery forever. That's why it's so important to choose a mate who provides you with more than momentary physical arousal, but rather an attraction based on intellectual, emotional, and spiritual compatibility as well. If a relationship gets to the point where you can predict everything your partner will do or say in a given situation, both in bed and out, it's time to start challenging and expanding your relationship.

The more I thought about this concept, the more I realized Charlie was right. Sex is the ideal forum for expanding the boundaries of a relationship. But to do that you need to be committed to communication and discovery. Most of us want to let go, to experience the world through fresh eyes, through each other's eyes, just like we did when we were children, to reawaken that youthful spirit, much like the White Tigress we talked about earlier on. But men, more than women, are trained from birth not to let go, to be responsible mature adults, to be bosses, husbands, protectors, providers, and fathers. Sex provides an outlet from the pressures of life's constraints.

Sex is the one place where, if there's enough love and trust in the other person's genuine desire, the sheer pleasure of letting go can be experienced in a concert of all the senses, which is not only sexually cathartic, but can be emotionally bonding in a way unparalleled by any other form of human interaction.

To achieve that, however, takes the kind of trust and understanding Charlie and his wife have. You have to be able to welcome the fact that there will always be more to explore, more fantasies that evolve. And the relationship must be strong enough to bend and grow without breaking.

"So that's your secret?" I asked Charlie.

He flashed me a mischievous grin. "Well, you know, we have other secrets too . . . sexy secrets. It's not like they're all kinky or anything; it's more the fact that they're things we know about each other that nobody else does: stuff we like to say or do that turns us on, fantasies we've never told anybody else. And I guess that's why no one in the world could ever come close to making me as hot as my wife does, even after all these years together. The truth is that when I think of something sexy, the first thing I want to do is tell her. Sex reminds me of my wife. And my wife reminds me of sex. And it all keeps on growing and expanding and twisting and turning in every direction, kind of like the universe. Take last night, for instance. . . ."

Then Charlie stopped himself. "Never mind; it's a secret."

Charlie stood up, still reeling from his memories of the night before. "Hey, I'm sorry to disappoint you, doc. I really don't have too much to say about particular positions and techniques. I guess from the outside looking in my sex life probably looks pretty normal and boring. . . . But, let me tell you something, I wouldn't trade one night with my wife for a year at the Playboy Mansion."

Charlie shut the door behind him.

I thought for a second about Einstein and his blunder of not recognizing that the universe was perpetually expanding.

My eye drifted to the photo of the Capilano Canyon Suspension Bridge on my desk.

Then I picked up the phone. "Hey, honey," I whispered into the phone "I have something I want to tell you. . . . It's sort of a secret. . . . Do you have a moment?"

"I do," she whispered, the two sexiest words in the English dictionary.

Bibliography

Angier, Natalie. *Woman, An Intimate Geography*. New York: Anchor, 1999.

Aron, Arthur, Elaine Aron, Colin McKenna, and Christina C. Norman. "Couples Shared Participation in Novel and Arousing Activities and Experienced Relationship Quality." *Journal of Personality and Social Psychology* Vol. 78, No. 2: 273–284 (2000).

Bechtel, Stefan, and Lawrence Roy Stain, (eds. of *Men's Health Magazine*). *Sex: A Man's Guide*. New York: Berkley, 1998.

Brooks, Gary R. *The Centerfold Syndrome*. New York: Josey-Bass, 1995.

Cambell, Keith, Craig A. Foster, Jeffrey D. Green, and Betty S. Witcher. "Arousal and Attraction: Evidence for Automatic and Controlled Process." *Journal of Personality and Social Psychology* Vol. 74, No. 1: 86–101 (1998).

Cattrall, Kim. *Satisfaction: Art of the Female Orgasm*. New York: Warner Books, 2003.

Cohen, Joseph. *The Penis Book*. New York: Broadway Books, 2004.

Comfort, Alex. *The Joy of Sex*. New York: Pocket Books, 1972.

Crenshaw, Theresa. *The Alchemy of Love and Lust*. New York: Pocket Books, 1997.

Fisher, Helen. *Why We Love*. New York: Henry Holt and Co., 2004.

Freud, Sigmund. *An Outline of Psychoanalysis*. New York: W. W. Norton, 1940.

Freud, Sigmund. *New Introductory Lectures on Psychoanalysis*. New York: W. W. Norton, 1940.

Furhman, Joel. *Eat to Live*. New York: Little, Brown, 2003.

Gottman, John. *The Seven Principles of Making Marriage Work*. New York: Three Rivers Press, 2001.

Herring, Richard. *Talking Cock*. New York: Thunder's Mouth Press 2004.

Kaplan, Helen Singer. *The Illustrated Manual of Sex Therapy*. New York: Brunner-Routledge, 1988.

Keesling, Barbara. *How to Make Love All Night*. New York: Harper Paperbacks, 1995.

Koedt, Anne. *The Myth of the Vaginal Orgasm*. New York: New York Radical Women, 1968.

Lai, Hsi. *The Sexual Teachings of the White Tigress*. Rochester, Vermont: Destiny Books, 2001.

Lamm, Steven. *The Hardness Factor*. New York: HarperCollins, 2005.

Leiblum, Sandra, and Raymond Rosen. *Principles and Practice of Sex Therapy, Third Edition*. New York: The Guilford Press, 2000.

Margolis, Jonathan. *O: The Intimate History of the Orgasm*. New York: Grove, 2004.

Masters, W. H., and V. E. Johnson. *Human Sexual Response*. Boston: Little, Brown, 1966.

Masters, W. H., and V. E. Johnson. *Human Sexual Inadequacy*. Boston: Little, Brown, 1970.

Money, John. *Love Maps*. New York: Prometheus Books, 1988

Morris, Desmond. *The Naked Woman*. New York: Thomas Dunne Books, 2005.

Rush, Norman. *Mortals*. New York: Knopf, 2003.

Schnarch, David. *Passionate Marriage*. New York: Owl Books, 1998.

Schultz, Louis R. *Out in the Open: The Complete Male Pelvis*. Berkeley, California: North Atlantic Books, 1999.

Tiger, Lionel. *The Decline of Males*. New York: St. Martins Press, 2000.

Tisdale, Sallie. *Talk Dirty to Me*. New York: Anchor Books, 1998.

Wellings, Kaye. *First Love, First Sex*. New York: HarperCollins, 1986.

Wiener-Davis, Michele. *The Sex-Starved Marriage*. New York: Simon and Schuster, 2003.

Acknowledgments

- Once again, I would like to thank my dear friend Naomi Pitcairn for her elegant illustrations, hysterical limericks, and extraordinary artistic eye.
- I am indebted to my friend, Sue Rosenstock, whose editorial insights greatly helped these pages.
- Many thanks to Judith Regan.
- Much appreciation goes to the editorial stewardship of Cassie Jones and everyone else on the Collins team for their support.
- My agent, Richard Abate, continually earns my appreciation for his strategic acumen and sound judgment.
- My Web site designer, Emily Blair, is to be cherished for her clean aesthetic, her lovely manner, and her incredible versatility.

- To my friend and mentor, Dr. William Granzig, I extend my heartfelt appreciation for his enthusiasm, wisdom, and humor, which are a constant source of intellectual rejuvenation.
- To everyone at AASECT (the American Association of Sex Educators, Counselors, and Therapists), thank you for your important work and for maintaining one of the liveliest online communities I've ever had the good fortune to participate in.
- To my wife, sons, family, and friends, words escape me: The ancient Greeks taught us six types of love—eros, ludus, storge, pragma, mania, and agape—and you've shown me the meaning of them all.
- And finally, I would like to thank the many men and women of all ages and backgrounds who were brave enough to share their innermost thoughts and feelings about sex with me. Thank you for your honesty and courage. As Hillel wrote, "If I am not for myself, then who will be for me? And if I am only for myself, then what am I? And if not now, when?"

BOOKS BY IAN KERNER, Ph.D.

SHE COMES FIRST
The Thinking Man's Guide to Pleasuring a Woman

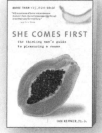

ISBN 978-0-06-053826-2 (paperback)

"Required reading for all men who are dating and all women who are wondering why they're not satisfied."
—Cindy Chupack, Writer/Executive Producer of *Sex and the City*

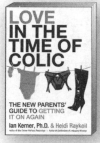

LOVE IN THE TIME OF COLIC
The New Parents' Guide to Getting It On Again

ISBN 978-0-06-146512-3 (paperback)

Funny and frank, *Love in the Time of Colic* will help parents take the charge out of this once-taboo subject, and put it back where it belongs—in the bedroom.

SEX RECHARGE
A Rejuvenation Plan for Couples and Singles

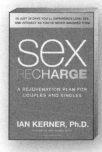

ISBN 978-0-06-123462-0 (paperback)

"Kerner makes intimacy intimate again, as well as downright lustful. You'll walk away trusting your instincts instead of subscribing to the fabricated ideas of what sexy 'should' be."
—Stephanie Klein, author of *Straight Up and Dirty*

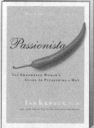

PASSIONISTA
The Empowered Woman's Guide to Pleasuring a Man

ISBN 978-0-06-083439-5 (paperback)

"*Passionista* satisfies the reader with tasty morsels of sexual enlightenment, nibble by nibble, bite by bite."
—Lou Paget, bestselling author of *How to Be a Great Lover*

BE HONEST—YOU'RE NOT THAT INTO HIM EITHER
Raise Your Standards and Reach for the Love You Deserve

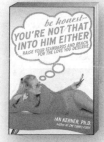

ISBN 978-0-06-083406-7 (paperback)

Kerner explores the battlefield of sex, hook-ups, go-nowhere relationships, and the dismal dating treadmill, simultaneously arming women with a sharper set of insights and the tools for change.

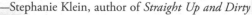